CW00972871

SITE-SPECIFIC CANCER SERIES

Prostate Cancer

Edited by
William P. Hogle, RN, MSN, OCN®

Oncology Nursing Society
Pittsburgh, Pennsylvania

ONS Publishing Division
Publisher: Leonard Mafrica, MBA, CAE
Director, Commercial Publishing/Technical Publications Editor: Barbara Sigler, RN, MNEd
Managing Editor: Lisa M. George, BA
Staff Editor: Amy Nicoletti, BA
Copy Editor: Laura Pinchot, BA
Graphic Designer: Dany Sjoen

Site-Specific Cancer Series: Prostate Cancer

Library of Congress Control Number: 2008942986

ISBN: 978-1-890504-77-9

Publisher's Note

Printed in the United States of America

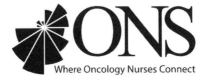

Oncology Nursing Society
Integrity • Innovation • Stewardship • Advocacy • Excellence • Inclusiveness

Contributors

Editor

William P. Hogle, RN, MSN, OCN®
Clinical Manager
UPMC Passavant Cancer Center
Pittsburgh, Pennsylvania
Chapter 3. Prostate Cancer Screening, Risk, Prevention, and Prognosis

Authors

Jormain O. Cady, ARNP, DNP(c), AOCN®
Nurse Practitioner, Radiation Oncology
Virginia Mason Medical Center
Seattle, Washington
Chapter 1. Overview; Chapter 2. Prostate Cancer Diagnosis and Staging

Cathy Fortenbaugh, RN, MSN, AOCN®
Oncology Clinical Nurse Specialist
Capital Health System
Trenton, New Jersey
Chapter 6. Survivorship Issues in Prostate Cancer

Tracy K. Gosselin, RN, MSN, PhD(c), AOCN®
Clinical Director, Oncology Services
Duke University Health System
Clinical Associate
Duke University School of Nursing
Durham, North Carolina
Chapter 7. Nursing Research Contributions to the Care of Patients With Prostate Cancer

Marilyn L. Haas, PhD, RN, CNS, ANP-C
Nurse Practitioner
Mountain Radiation Oncology
Asheville, North Carolina
Chapter 4. Treatment Modalities for Prostate Cancer

Susan Moore, RN, MSN, ANP, AOCN®
Oncology Nurse Practitioner/Consultant
Cancer Expertise
Chicago, Illinois
Chapter 5. Nursing Implications of Prostate Cancer

Linda Reuber, RN-BC, MSN, CHTC, AOCNS®
Oncology Clinical Nurse Specialist
Renown Regional Medical Center
Reno, Nevada
Chapter 1. Overview

Sarah Yenser Wood, RN, MSN, ANP, AOCNP®
Genitourinary Oncology Nurse Practitioner
Duke University Medical Center
Durham, North Carolina
Chapter 4. Treatment Modalities for Prostate Cancer

Contents

Foreword

You have cancer. These are the words I heard, but didn't believe, as they were spoken by my doctor. As a 43-year-old (I still consider this young) oncology sales representative, I found it incredibly ironic that I was selling therapy for prostate cancer at the time I found out that I had it. Fortunately, I was diagnosed early enough that four years after surgery and radiation, I am here to write the foreword to this book. When I was first asked to be involved in this project, it was my experience as a prostate cancer survivor that was thought to be important and worthy of putting pen to paper. Instead, I would like to write about what nurses mean to me and to so many who have heard the words "You have prostate cancer."

I have a somewhat unique perspective in that oncology nurses are my customers who I see every day in my job. Now that I am a cancer survivor, they are so much more to me than customers. Like most male patients with a serious illness, I was scared and alone in my fear as I pretended to be in control. The first person I met before my oncologist came in the room was my nurse. She looked me right in the eye, gently put her arm on my shoulder, and simply said, "We're going to take good care of you." For the first time, I felt like I was going to be OK. My oncology nurse started me on my journey to survivorship. I don't want to underestimate the value of my physicians, but I can't overestimate the value of my nurses. It was a memorable day and a memorable statement—at last, someone made me feel at ease.

Highlighted in this book is the important role of the nurse in caring for men who are at risk for or are living with prostate cancer. The oncology nurse's role includes the many aspects of education and prevention, and detection and treatment, as well as assisting with survivorship issues and taking part in nursing research. This comprehensive resource provides nurses and other healthcare professionals with essential information for their practice, which ultimately will benefit many patients with prostate cancer and their caregivers.

On behalf of all men with prostate cancer who journey through diagnosis and treatment with our eyes aimed at survivorship, this message is for you:

We appreciate your caring smile and your gentle touch. Thanks for being the consummate professional in all you do as you put up with big babies like me. Thanks for the hugs and the tough love and for giving an emotional shove. The poking and prodding is part of the game, but you always make us laugh as we struggle and strain. You are a nurse, knowledgeable and well trained to help us in our plight, and we will never forget you as we continue the fight.

You are an oncology nurse; you constantly impress. You and thousands among ONS!

Thomas J. Doré
Senior Oncology Sales Consultant
Prostate Cancer Survivor
Pittsburgh, PA

CHAPTER 1

Overview

Linda Reuber, RN-BC, MSN, CHTC, AOCNS®, and Jormain O. Cady, ARNP, DNP(c), AOCN®

Introduction

With the exception of skin cancer, prostate cancer is the most commonly diagnosed cancer in the United States and is the second most lethal cancer among men. Approximately 186,320 new cases are estimated to be diagnosed in 2008, and the disease accounts for roughly 10% of cancer-related deaths in men. The lifetime risk of developing prostate cancer is one out of six, and nearly 30,000 men die yearly from this disease (American Cancer Society [ACS], 2008; Jemal et al., 2008). These statistics reinforce the ongoing need for further research into all aspects of the disease, including successful treatment outcomes. Multidisciplinary collaboration among urology, radiation oncology, medical oncology, and nursing is imperative, as attempts to improve outcomes and quality of life persist. In addition to multidisciplinary collaboration, funding for prostate cancer research and patient support is paramount in the progress toward cure.

The National Cancer Institute (NCI) estimated that $309 million in 2006 and $305.6 million in 2007 were spent on prostate cancer research. In contrast, proposed funding for breast, colorectal, and lung cancer research was $551.1 million, $249.1 million, and $261.9 million, respectively (NCI, 2006). An additional estimate for the annual cost of prostate cancer treatment is approximately $8 billion (NCI, 2007). Despite significant expenditure of resources, prostate cancer remains the second leading cause of cancer death among men, behind only lung cancer (Jemal et al., 2008).

Numerous organizations aim to increase awareness of prostate cancer and advocate for increased federal spending. These organizations serve as portals of information and provide support for patients, caregivers, laypersons, and professional healthcare providers. The mission of the National Prostate Cancer Coalition (2005) is to rapidly reduce the burden of prostate cancer on American men and their families through awareness, outreach, and advocacy. The Prostate Cancer Foundation (n.d.), the world's largest philanthropic source of support for prostate cancer research, focuses on improving treatments and finding a cure for recurrent prostate cancer. A number of other nonprofit prostate cancer groups exist, including the American Cancer Society, the Prostate Cancer Education Council, Us TOO International Prostate Cancer Education and Support Network, and the Prostate Cancer Research Institute. All of these groups offer a wealth of information on prostate cancer awareness as well as ongoing financial and emotional support to those afflicted with the disease. The alliance among various nonprofit organizations, advocacy groups, and professional medical societies continues to advance the knowledge and treatment of prostate cancer, along with dissemination of vital information.

A number of professional medical organizations also are keenly interested in and support the fight against prostate cancer. The annual Prostate Cancer Symposium is a collaborative effort of the American Society of Clinical Oncology, the American Society for Therapeutic Radiology and Oncology, the Society of Urologic Oncology, and the Prostate Cancer Foundation. The annual meetings cover numerous topics, including updates on epidemiology, risk factors, prevention, screening and diagnosis, and treatment, including novel treatment approaches. The research and abstracts presented at these meetings illustrate the significant challenge in fully understanding and treating prostate cancer.

Epidemiology

Cancer epidemiology is the study of cancer patterns in populations and cancer causation. Through epidemiologic studies, a greater understanding of changing patterns of cancer incidence and mortality, risk factors, prevention strategies, and the role of genetic variation in cancer etiology has been gained (Tucker, 2001). The epidemiology of prostate cancer has been notoriously difficult to study, making the disease a formidable challenge to practitioners and epidemiologists (Boyle, Severi, & Giles, 2003). The disease is prevalent and has considerable morbidity and mortality, yet the etiology remains elusive. Advancing age, race, and family history are the only definitive risk factors, although genetic variables also have been suggested to comprise more than 40% of risk factors (Hsing & Chokkalingam, 2006). Men with a first-degree relative diagnosed with prostate cancer have a twofold greater risk of developing prostate cancer compared to men without a family history of the disease (ACS, 2007). African American men clearly have higher incidence and mortality rates for prostate cancer. In addition, African American men often present with a higher stage of cancer and, as a result, die at a younger age from the disease (Jayadevappa, Chhatre, Weiner, Bloom, & Malkowicz, 2005). Some theorized risk factors include androgenic hormones, diet, chronic inflammation, and vitamin D, all of which are currently under study (Hsing & Chokkalingam). The Cohort Consortium is a collaborative effort with multiple study groups evaluating large numbers of individuals with prostate cancer. Launched in 2003, the consortium's primary intent is to evaluate genetic influences and their association with prostate cancer (NCI, 2008).

The Surveillance, Epidemiology, and End Results (SEER) Program of NCI collects and maintains the most comprehensive information regarding the epidemiology of prostate cancer. The SEER database (http://seer.cancer.gov) is the largest database in the United States and Europe. The SEER program, established in 1973 as part of NCI, collects cancer incidence, treatment, and survival data, which are used to monitor the impact of cancer on the U.S. population. Eleven SEER geographic areas maintain population-based cancer reporting systems, including the states of Connecticut, Hawaii, Iowa, New Mexico, and Utah and the metropolitan areas of Atlanta, Detroit, Los Angeles, San Francisco-Oakland, San Jose-Monterey, and Seattle-Puget Sound. These regions cover approximately 14% of the total U.S. population and were selected to provide information from diverse population subgroups, such as racial and ethnic groups and urban and rural residents (Stanford et al., 1999).

Additional information regarding epidemiology as it relates to incidence and mortality of prostate cancer can be found in Chapter 2.

Anatomy and Physiology

The term *prostate* was originally derived from the Greek word *prohistani*, meaning "to stand in front of," and has been attributed to Herophilus of Alexandria, who used the term in 335 BC to describe the organ located in front of the urinary bladder. Although previously described, detailed anatomic depictions of the prostate gland did not appear until the Renaissance period of world history (AD 1400–1600) (Kirby, Christmas, & Brawer, 2001).

The prostate is a firm, partly glandular and partly muscular structure located within the lower pelvis immediately below the internal urethral orifice and around the beginning

of the urethra (see Figures 1-1 and 1-2). Essentially shaped like a walnut, the gland is situated below the inferior part of the pubic symphysis, above the deep layer of the urogenital diaphragm and in front of the rectum, through which it may

---

Figure 1-1. Anterior View of the Prostate Located at the Base of the Urinary Bladder

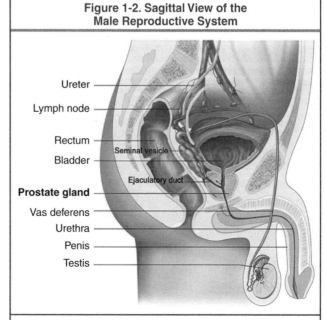

Labels: Ureter, Lymph node, Rectum, Bladder, **Prostate gland**, Vas deferens, Urethra, Penis, Testis

Note. Illustration created by Terese Winslow; used courtesy of the National Cancer Institute.

Figure 1-2. Sagittal View of the Male Reproductive System

Labels: Ureter, Lymph node, Rectum, Bladder, **Prostate gland**, Vas deferens, Urethra, Penis, Testis, Seminal vesicle, Ejaculatory duct

Note. Illustration created by Terese Winslow; used courtesy of the National Cancer Institute.

be palpated, especially when enlarged (Gray, 1985). Palpation of the prostate gland is included as part of a digital rectal examination (DRE) and is considered an essential component of screening for prostate cancer. Because of its anatomic location, DRE is useful in detecting palpable abnormalities in the posterior and lateral aspects of the prostate gland (see inset of Figure 1-3).

The anatomic size of a normal, nonmalignant prostate gland is 28–47 cubic centimeters and is dependent on age (Bosch, Tilling, Bohnen, Bangma, & Donovan, 2007). The

---

Figure 1-3. The Prostate and Nearby Organs

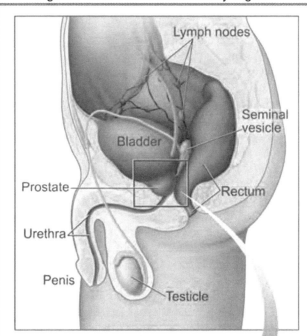

This shows the prostate and nearby organs.

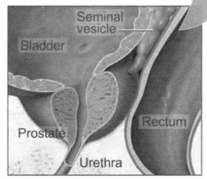

This shows the inside of the prostate, urethra, rectum, and bladder.

Portions of the prostate gland are palpable via digital rectal examination because of its proximity to the distal rectum.

Note. Illustrations created by Alan Hoofring; used courtesy of the National Cancer Institute.

---

prostate, seminal vesicles, and bulbourethral glands (glands of Cowper) constitute the accessory glands of reproduction. The primary function of the prostate is to secrete seminal fluids that act as a medium for spermatozoa during ejaculation. The prostatic secretion constitutes the first and major portion of the ejaculate, with the seminal vesicle contributing a small terminal amount.

The prostate gland consists of four anatomic zones: the peripheral, central, transition, and fibromuscular zones. The peripheral zone in the normal gland comprises about 75% of the entire prostate. This zone stretches from the apex to the base and covers the bottom and wraps around the sides of the gland. The next largest zone is the central zone, which constitutes the majority of the prostate base. The ejaculatory ducts are located within the central zone space. The transition zone, comprising 5%–10% of the gland in young men, is divided into two separate lobules on either side of the prostatic urethra. The outermost zone, the anterior fibromuscular zone, consists mostly of smooth muscle (Applewhite, Matlaga, McCullough, & Hall, 2001). In regard to general prostate disease, the development of benign prostatic hypertrophy (BPH) typically occurs in the transition zone, whereas 75% of malignant disease develops in the peripheral zone but may invade all three zones (Applewhite et al.). Prostate cancer within the transition zone often can be felt by DRE as a nodular or indurated presentation (Carroll, Lee, Fuks, & Kantoff, 2001).

A capsule or membrane surrounds the prostate, simply called the prostatic capsule. Outside the capsule lies a fascial sheath, which contains nerves and lymphatics, and the prostatic plexus. The neurovascular bundles responsible for producing an erection are located outside of Denonvillier's fascia, which is the rectovesical septum. Increased understanding of the fascia and neurovascular bundles has led to a change in the conventional approach to surgical excision of the gland. Refined surgical techniques now allow for the nerve bundles to remain intact, thus reducing postoperative impotence (Reiter & deKernion, 2002). Additional information about surgical treatment for prostate cancer, including a nerve-sparing approach, can be found in Chapter 4.

Screening for Prostate Cancer

Aggressive prostate-specific antigen (PSA) screening programs over the past few years have resulted in increased detection of early-stage cancers and a decreased number of patients presenting with metastatic disease, and possibly have reduced prostate cancer–related mortality (Ekman, Adolfsson, & Gronberg, 1999; Tarone, Chu, & Brawley, 2000). Approximately 75% of men older than age 50 have participated in prostate cancer screening in the United States (Sirovich, Schwartz, & Woloshin, 2003). Common prostate cancers generally are slow growing, but some can be biologically aggressive. The lifetime risk of a prostate cancer diagnosis in males is 18%, whereas the lifetime risk of dying from prostate cancer is approximately 3% (Kramer & Siroky, 2004; Thompson & Ankerst, 2007). Given the prevalence of clinically insignificant prostate cancers, reducing the costs and morbidity related to overdetection, diagnostic procedures for benign disease, and overtreatment is important to consider.

ACS (2007) recommends annual DRE and PSA screening in men older than age 50 who have a life expectancy of at least 10 years. Screening for men at higher risk for prostate cancer (African Americans or those with a first-degree relative with a prostate cancer diagnosis before age 65) should be offered at 45 years of age. Prostate cancer screening programs continue to expand in the United States although controversy about the benefits of population screening still persist and a strong consensus regarding appropriate screening practice cannot be agreed upon. Lack of strong supporting evidence has led other countries, such as Canada and the United Kingdom, to forgo recommendations for systematic screening programs (Templeton, 2007; Thompson & Ankerst, 2007; Turner, 2007). Although evidence has shown increased numbers of early prostate cancers diagnosed in populations with broad-based screening programs, the clinical significance of these cancers is unclear, and systematic reviews have failed to identify a mortality benefit related to PSA screening (Harris & Lohr, 2002; Ilic, O'Connor, Green, & Wilt, 2007).

Presentation of Disease

Early-stage prostate cancer, like other early-stage malignancies, may be present in the absence of significant or noticeable symptoms, which highlights the necessity of ongoing screening for at-risk populations. Serum PSA levels may or may not be elevated in the presence of early disease. However, in the majority of men diagnosed with prostate cancer, a PSA level will exceed the normal range of 0–4 ng/ml. Age- and race-specific PSA values are discussed in greater detail in Chapter 2. DRE also may yield little beneficial information as to the presence of early disease, as only a portion of the gland is palpable by even the most experienced clinician.

Upon confirmation of prostate cancer and retrospective consideration, the patient may acknowledge that some symptoms such as frequency, urgency, and nocturia have been present but that he viewed them as simply bothersome and did not mention. As prostate cancer progresses beyond the early stage, urinary symptoms such as decreased stream, increased frequency, and difficulty starting or maintaining stream may develop. However, these same symptoms are present with BPH. Some men may present with hematuria, hematospermia, infection, or varying degrees of impotence. In advanced disease, patients may present with bowel or bladder incontinence, motor weakness, peripheral neuropathy, leg edema, or varying degrees of bone pain. Although treatment modalities vary, the stage of disease upon presentation significantly influences the overall course of treatment. See Chapter 4 for an in-depth examination of treatment options for prostate cancer.

Patterns of Metastasis and Progression of Disease

Most prostate cancers are considered to be very treatable, and in the absence of metastatic disease, cure is possible (Schlomm, Erbersdobler, Mirlacher, & Sauter, 2007). However, even in the presence of metastatic disease, prostate cancer may be controlled for extended periods of time. Mean survival with metastatic disease has been reported as 3–3.5 years, with 4–6-year survival expectations for those with minimal metastatic disease burden (Ekman et al., 1999). Historically, hormonal agents and chemotherapy are used most often in patients with metastatic disease to preserve quality of life and prolong survival (Petrylak et al., 2004).

Dominant theories for the process of metastatic disease in prostate cancer include the *mechanical theory* and *seed-and-soil theory*. The mechanical theory describes direct extension of tumor and spread through the regional lymphatic system into the lumbar spine. The seed-and-soil theory proposes the presence of specific factors that contribute to preferential growth in certain tissues (including the bone, lung, liver, and adrenals). Therefore, while cancer cells may widely disseminate throughout the body, preferential growth in bone may occur because of tissue-specific environmental characteristics that create a favorable condition for growth.

Local/regional disease control appears to decrease the risk of dissemination and metastasis. Biochemical recurrence (increasing PSA level) following surgery or definitive radiation therapy may represent biochemical recurrence only or local/regional recurrence in the prostate or prostate bed. Radiographic imaging often is obtained but may be of limited utility in defining actual disease involvement in this setting. Although up to one-third of patients with biochemical recurrence after prostatectomy may have distant disease, the likelihood of a positive bone scan if the PSA level is less than 7 ng/ml is low and therefore not warranted unless bone symptoms are present (Han et al., 2003). Salvage local therapy (with or without systemic hormonal intervention) often is indicated in this situation to offer greater benefit of local control.

The most frequent sites of metastatic involvement in prostate cancer are the lymph nodes and bone, but liver and lung metastasis also may occur (Gomez, Manoharan, Kim, & Soloway, 2004). Metastatic nodal involvement (occurring outside of the true pelvis) often progresses in a stepwise fashion with local spread to pelvic nodes followed by retroperitoneal and mediastinal adenopathy (Hricak, Choyke, Eberhardt, Leibel, & Scardino, 2007). Patterns of bone metastasis classically demonstrate multiple small, occasionally congruent, metastatic lesions typically involving the axial skeleton

(Buscombe & Hilson, 1999). Bone metastasis from prostate cancer can appear as osteoblastic or osteolytic lesions. These lesions usually can be seen on a plain x-ray film, or correlation with a radionuclide bone scan may be necessary. Bony lesions may or may not be painful, and treatment usually is withheld unless pain is present or an eminent risk of fracture exists, especially to a weight-bearing bone. Solitary metastatic lesions in prostate cancer are less common, but when they occur, they often involve the pelvis or lumbar spine. Late disease often is characterized by involvement of the majority of the axial skeleton and proximal femurs or humeri as well as distant organs such as lung and brain. Generally, this is accompanied by significant increases in serum PSA levels.

Conclusion

Prostate cancer is a relatively common malignancy in the United States that poses significant challenges to public health. As the baby boomer population continues to age, the incidence and prevalence of this disease will increase, further straining the present healthcare system. Prostate cancer is considered a slow-growing disease and may remain indolent for many years prior to diagnosis. Unlike many other primary malignancies, prostate cancer continues to be effectively treated by numerous modalities. Nurses who care for patients with prostate cancer must remain abreast of the multiple treatment options available as well as the morbidity associated with each modality. In addition, nurses should be active in prostate cancer education and early detection programs. Such involvement assists patients, families, and communities in better understanding the benefits and controversies surrounding prostate cancer screening and management.

Subsequent chapters of this text are meant to provide nurses with detailed knowledge regarding the detection, staging, and treatment of prostate cancer. In addition, management of treatment-related side effects, survivorship, and nursing research issues also are explored.

References

American Cancer Society. (2007). *What are the risks factors for prostate cancer?* Retrieved March 6, 2008, from http://www.cancer.org/docroot/CRI/content/CRI_2_4_2X_What_are_the_risk_factors_for_prostate_cancer_36.asp?sitearea=

American Cancer Society. (2008). *Cancer facts and figures, 2008.* Retrieved June 9, 2008, from http://www.cancer.org/downloads/STT/2008CAFFfinalsecured.pdf

Applewhite, J.C., Matlaga, B.R., McCullough, D.L., & Hall, M.C. (2001). Transrectal ultrasound and biopsy in the early diagnosis of prostate cancer. *Cancer Control, 8*(2), 141–150.

Bosch, J.L., Tilling, K., Bohnen, A.M., Bangma, C.H., & Donovan, J.L. (2007). Establishing normal reference ranges for prostate volume change with age in the population-based Krimpen-study: Prediction of future prostate volume in individual men. *Prostate, 67*(16), 1816–1824.

Boyle, P., Severi, G., & Giles, G.G. (2003). The epidemiology of prostate cancer. *Urologic Clinics of North America, 30*(2), 209–217.

Buscombe, J., & Hilson, A. (1999). Nuclear medicine in prostate cancer. In A.V. Kaisary, G.P. Murphy, L. Denis, & K. Griffiths (Eds.), *Textbook of prostate cancer pathology, diagnosis and treatment* (pp. 157–167). Malden, MA: Blackwell Science.

Carroll, P.R., Lee, K.L., Fuks, Z.Y., & Kantoff, P.W. (2001). Cancer of the prostate. In V.T. Devita, Jr., S. Hellman, & S.A. Rosenberg (Eds.), *Cancer: Principles and practice of oncology* (6th ed., pp. 1418–1479). Philadelphia: Lippincott Williams & Wilkins.

Ekman, P., Adolfsson, J., & Gronberg, H. (1999). The natural history of prostate cancer. In A.V. Kaisary, G.P. Murphy, L. Denis, & K. Griffiths (Eds.), *Textbook of prostate cancer pathology, diagnosis and treatment* (pp. 1–16). Malden, MA: Blackwell Science.

Gomez, P., Manoharan, M., Kim, S.S., & Soloway, M.S. (2004). Radionuclide bone scintigraphy in patients with biochemical recurrence after radical prostatectomy: When is it indicated? *BJU International, 94*(3), 299–302.

Gray, H. (1985). The urogenital system: Male genital organs. In C.D. Clemente (Ed.), *Anatomy of the human body* (30th ed., pp. 1564–1566). Philadelphia: Lea & Febiger.

Han, M., Partin, A.W., Zahurac, M., Piantadosi, S., Epstein, J.I., & Walsh, P.C. (2003). Biochemical (prostate specific antigen) recurrence probability following radical prostatectomy for clinically localized prostate cancer. *Journal of Urology, 169*(2), 517–523.

Harris, R., & Lohr, K.N. (2002). Screening for prostate cancer: An update of the evidence for the U.S. Preventive Services Task Force. *Annals of Internal Medicine, 137*(11), 917–929.

Hricak, H., Choyke, P.L., Eberhardt, S.C., Leibel, S.A., & Scardino, P.T. (2007). Imaging prostate cancer: Multidisciplinary perspective. *Radiology, 243*(1), 28–53.

Hsing, A.W., & Chokkalingam, A.P. (2006). Prostate cancer epidemiology. *Frontiers in Bioscience, 11,* 1388–1413.

Ilic, D., O'Connor, D., Green, S., & Wilt, T. (2007). Screening for prostate cancer: A Cochrane systematic review. *Cancer Causes and Control, 18*(3), 279–285.

Jayadevappa, R., Chhatre, S., Weiner, M., Bloom, B.S., & Malkowicz, S.B. (2005). Medical care cost of patients with prostate cancer. *Urologic Oncology, 23*(3), 155–162.

Jemal, A., Siegel, R., Ward, E., Hao, Y., Xu, J., Murray, T., et al. (2008). Cancer statistics, 2008. *CA: A Cancer Journal for Clinicians, 58*(2), 71–96.

Kirby, R.S., Christmas, T.J., & Brawer, M.K. (2001). *Prostate cancer* (2nd ed.). London: Mosby.

Kramer, A., & Siroky, M.B. (2004). Neoplasms of the genitourinary tract. In M.B. Siroky, R.D. Oates, & R.K. Babayan (Eds.), *Handbook of urology: Diagnosis and therapy* (3rd ed., pp. 249–300). Philadelphia: Lippincott Williams & Wilkins.

National Cancer Institute. (2006, May 19). *Fact sheet: Cancer research funding.* Retrieved June 4, 2006, from http://www.cancer.gov/cancertopics/factsheet/NCI/research-funding

National Cancer Institute. (2007). *A snapshot of prostate cancer.* Retrieved March 6, 2008, from http://planning.cancer.gov/disease/Prostate-Snapshot.pdf

National Cancer Institute. (2008, March 31). *Breast and prostate cancer and hormone-related gene variant study.* Retrieved June 4, 2008, from http://www.epi.grants.cancer.gov/BPC3

National Prostate Cancer Coalition. (2005). *Public policy platform: Prostate cancer advocacy goals for 2006/fiscal year 2007.* Retrieved June 4, 2006, from http://www.fightprostatecancer.org/site/PageServer?pagename=Fullpage_FY07platform

Petrylak, D.P., Tangen, C.M., Hussain, M.H., Lara, P.N., Jones, J.A., Taplin, M.E., et al. (2004). Docetaxel and estramustine compared with mitoxantrone and prednisone for advanced refractory prostate cancer. *New England Journal of Medicine, 351*(15), 1513–1520.

Prostate Cancer Foundation. (n.d.). *About the Prostate Cancer Foundation.* Retrieved March 6, 2008, from http://www.prostatecancerfoundation.org/site/c.itIWK2OSG/b.46632/k.E3BA/About_PCF.htm

Reiter, R.E., & deKernion, J.B. (2002). Epidemiology, etiology, and prevention of prostate cancer. In P.C. Walsh (Ed.), *Campbell's urology* (8th ed., pp. 3003–3019). Philadelphia: Saunders.

Schlomm, T., Erbersdobler, A., Mirlacher, M., & Sauter, G. (2007). Molecular staging of prostate cancer in the year 2007. *World Journal of Urology, 25*(1), 19–30.

Sirovich, B.E., Schwartz, L.M., & Woloshin, S. (2003). Screening men for prostate and colorectal cancer in the United States: Does practice reflect the evidence? *JAMA, 289*(11), 1414–1420.

Stanford, J.L., Stephenson, R.A., Coyle, L.M., Cerhan, J., Correa, R., Eley, J.W., et al. (Eds.). (1999). *Prostate cancer trends, 1973–1995, SEER program, National Cancer Institute* [NIH Publication No. 99-4543]. Bethesda, MD: National Cancer Institute.

Tarone, R.E., Chu, K.C., & Brawley, O.W. (2000). Implications of stage-specific survival rates in assessing recent declines in prostate cancer mortality rates. *Epidemiology, 11*(2), 167–170.

Templeton, H. (2007). Prostate cancer—presentation, diagnosis and treatment: What does the literature say? *International Journal of Urological Nursing, 1*(1), 6–17.

Thompson, I.M., & Ankerst, D.P. (2007). Prostate-specific antigen in the early detection of prostate cancer. *Canadian Medical Association Journal, 176*(13), 1853–1858.

Tucker, M.A. (2001). Epidemiology of cancer. In V.T. DeVita, Jr., S. Hellman, & S.A. Rosenberg (Eds.), *Cancer: Principles and practice of oncology* (6th ed., pp. 219–228). Philadelphia: Lippincott Williams & Williams.

Turner, B. (2007). Diagnosis and treatment of patients with prostate cancer: The nurse's role. *Nursing Standard, 21*(39), 48–56.

CHAPTER 2

Prostate Cancer Diagnosis and Staging

Jormain O. Cady, ARNP, DNP(c), AOCN®

Introduction

Prostate cancer is a disease that may manifest itself in a broad spectrum of ways, with marked variability in natural history (ranging from the clinically insignificant to high metastatic potential). Assessment of tumor characteristics and staging will guide the treatment recommendations, which may range from observation only (active surveillance or "watchful waiting") to multimodality intervention. Understanding the anatomic and biologic staging of prostate cancer is essential to understanding how selection of therapeutic options is made and provides a basis from which to help patients place their diagnosis in context. Surgery, radiation therapy, and hormonal therapy (androgen deprivation therapy) have been the mainstays of prostate cancer treatment. Chemotherapy also may be warranted in some instances, including advanced disease. Treatment modalities may be used alone or in combination, depending on histologic review, disease stage, patients' overall health condition, life expectancy, and preferences.

Incidence and Mortality

Prostate cancer is common among males, and incidence has been steadily increasing in the United States over the past several years. In the United States, more than 186,320 new cases of prostate cancer are estimated to be diagnosed in 2008, with approximately 28,660 estimated deaths (Jemal et al., 2008). For men, it is the most commonly encountered noncutaneous cancer diagnosis and second leading cause of cancer-related death, with lung cancer being the first.

The incidence of prostate cancer increases with advancing age and rarely occurs in men younger than 40. Autopsy studies have documented the presence of prostate cancer in 15%–30% of men older than age 50, with the incidence risk doubling per decade of life. Factors that cause prostate cancer to be clinically significant in some men but not others are yet unknown. Other risks include African American

ethnicity, family history of prostate cancer, and abnormal digital rectal examination (DRE) (Thompson et al., 2006) (see Figure 2-1). Hispanic ethnicity and history of prior negative prostate biopsy are associated with reduced prostate cancer risk. In a subanalysis of 5,519 men in the placebo group of the Prostate Cancer Prevention Trial, end-of-study biopsies indicated predictors of high-grade disease at time of diagnosis to be abnormal DRE, history of prior prostate biopsy, African American race, older age, and an increase in prostate-specific antigen (PSA) velocity (degree of interval PSA increase) (Thompson et al., 2006).

In addition to being disproportionately diagnosed with prostate cancer, African Americans also bear the burden of increased mortality. This may, in part, be the result of limited access to and utilization of health services among African American communities. Evidence has shown that the relatively

---

Figure 2-1. Prostate Cancer Risk Factors

Probable
- Diet (high fat)
- Ethnicity/race
- Positive family history
- Hormones (elevated testosterone/dihydrotestosterone)
- Obesity
- Older age
- Prostatic intraepithelial neoplasia
- Sedentary lifestyle

Potential
- Alcohol
- Environmental exposures (i.e., cadmium)
- Industrial/occupational exposures
- Sexual activity
- Smoking
- Socioeconomic factors
- Vasectomy
- Viruses and infections

Note. Based on information from Bostwick et al., 2004.

recent publication of national prostate cancer diagnosis and staging guidelines (National Comprehensive Cancer Network [NCCN], American Urological Association, and American College of Radiology [ACR]) in 1995 appears to have resulted in more appropriate prostate cancer care for most men across the board and thus contributed to some degree in reducing the amount of racial disparities in care encountered (Abraham, Wan, Montagnet, Wong, & Armstrong, 2007).

Diagnosis

Most prostate cancers are initially diagnosed following presentation with an abnormal PSA value, often performed for screening purposes (Thompson et al., 2006). Abnormal DRE also will prompt further investigation, including prostate biopsy. On occasion, prostate cancer may be diagnosed as an incidental finding on pathologic review following a transurethral resection of the prostate, which may have been performed initially for benign reasons.

Relatively few patients present with symptoms specifically related to prostate cancer or metastatic disease. Obstructive urinary symptoms (e.g., urinary frequency, nocturia, decreased urinary stream, incomplete urinary emptying) may be present at diagnosis but are not specific to prostate cancer and frequently are associated with benign prostatic hypertrophy (BPH). Other symptoms that may be present include hematuria, hematospermia, or erectile dysfunction (Turner, 2007). New-onset erectile dysfunction should prompt consideration of a possible prostate cancer diagnosis (or other prostate pathology), as erectile function depends on input from the neurovascular bundle within the periprostatic tissue, which is subject to impingement in the presence of an enlarged gland. Back, hip, or other bone pain from metastatic disease is a late finding and less frequently is a presenting symptom of prostate cancer, particularly in areas where systematic screening occurs.

Evaluation of serum PSA level, whether obtained for screening purposes or clinical suspicion of prostate cancer, is an essential component of prostate cancer diagnosis. PSA is a glycoprotein responsible for liquefying semen and is produced almost exclusively by the prostate gland. Active PSA (binds to protein) is converted to inactive PSA (remains non–protein bound) within the prostate and generally enters circulation in this form (*free PSA*). Serum PSA testing measures both protein-bound (*complexed PSA*) and free PSA, resulting in the *total PSA*. Therefore, PSA is specific to the prostate rather than to prostate cancer itself, often complicating interpretation because of the low volume of prostate cancer proportionally compared with normal healthy prostate tissue in early-stage prostate cancers. Although an elevated serum PSA level increases the likelihood that prostate cancer is present, the specificity of PSA testing as a marker is not optimal. Other factors, such as BPH or prostate inflammation or infection,

also can result in abnormally elevated PSA levels. An abnormal PSA value cannot reliably distinguish prostate cancer from benign sources of PSA elevation.

Many modifications to PSA evaluation and related tests have been investigated in an effort to improve the positive predictive value of PSA screening (see Table 2-1). Prostate malignancy affects the permeability of the basement membrane and allows escape of PSA precursors and related kallikreins (pro-PSA, human glandular kallikrein, and complexed PSA). Research suggests that detection of these biomarkers may correlate with greater likelihood of malignancy and aid in diagnosis when performed in combination with PSA testing (Vickers et al., 2007). However, to date, appropriate utilization of these biomarkers and interpretation must still be made with caution.

Although a PSA level greater than 4 ng/ml commonly is considered abnormal, prostate cancer has been identified in approximately 15% of men with screening PSA levels less than 4 ng/ml (Thompson et al., 2004), thus prompting greater consideration of the criteria for prostate biopsy. PSA level therefore should be considered as a continuous (rather than dichotomous) biomarker for prostate cancer. "Normal" levels (0–4 ng/ml) do not necessarily correlate with absolute lack of cancer, and diagnosis in these men is important, as organ-confined disease (and therefore curable disease) is more common when the PSA level is low. The index of cancer suspicion rises with higher PSA values. In men with no other risk factors, the risk of positive prostate biopsy increases with rising PSA levels.

Researchers have investigated characteristics that help to identify correlations with greater likelihood of positive biopsy associated with PSA values. Rate of change in PSA values over time, including *PSA doubling time* (PSADT) and *PSA velocity* (PSAV), have been associated with increased risk of adverse clinical outcomes (metastatic disease and prostate-specific mortality) after initial treatment for prostate cancer. Unfortunately, evidence has not determined that they are important predictors of positive prostate biopsy in undiagnosed men (even when suspicion of prostate cancer is present based on exam findings) because of the natural variation of PSA levels in the normal population when PSA level is relatively low (less than 10 ng/ml) (Spurgeon et al., 2007). Attempts to estimate the risk of positive prostate biopsy based on age, family history, current PSA level, and DRE findings have been investigated and may assist in identifying those who have a clinically significant risk for developing prostate cancer (positive predictive value of 25%) with PSA screening results of less than 4 ng/ml (Thompson et al., 2006).

Another study of 2,700 men undergoing prostate biopsy found that age, DRE findings, and free-to-total PSA ratio were the greatest predictors of a positive biopsy, although inclusion of other risk factors (such as ethnicity, family history of prostate cancer, and presence of urinary symptoms) increased the sensitivity (Nam et al., 2007). Use of such additional information

Table 2-1. Prostate-Specific Antigen (PSA) Studies Used When Evaluating Prostate Cancer

PSA Studies	Normal Values	Purpose	Clinical Significance
Total PSA (tPSA)	0–4 ng/ml	Total serum PSA value (free and protein-bound PSA)	tPSA is used for primary screening and recurrence monitoring after treatment. It may be elevated in benign prostate hypertrophy, prostate cancer, prostate inflammation, and perineal trauma.
Free PSA (fPSA)	> 15%–25%	PSA is converted from active (binds to protein) to inactive (remains non–protein bound) in the prostate. Prostate cancer is associated with disruption of the basement membrane, allowing greater access of active PSA into the serum. Free PSA represents the percentage of non–protein bound (inactive) serum PSA.	Lower percentage of fPSA is more suggestive of prostate cancer versus benign source of PSA elevation.
Free-to-total PSA ratio (F/T PSA)	< 15%	Represents the ratio of unbound PSA to total PSA (bound and unbound) in the serum	F/T PSA ratio is reduced in prostate cancer.
Complexed PSA (cPSA)	0–3.75 ng/ml	Measurement of serum PSA bound to specific proteins	Marginal improvement occurs in specificity with addition of cPSA levels to tPSA.
PSA density (PSAD)	< 0.15 ng/ml/cm^3	Relationship of the PSA level to prostate volume (PSA divided by prostate volume)	Higher PSAD is associated with increased risk of cancer but is not as predictive as free-PSA.
PSA velocity	Increase of greater than 0.35–0.75 ng/ml/year	Measurement of rate of PSA increase over time	Higher PSA velocity is associated with increased risk of malignancy.
Pro-PSA	Not established	Precursor hormone produced and converted to PSA in the prostate.	Presence of serum pro-PSA more commonly is associated with malignancy than benign prostate conditions.
Age-specific PSA ranges	40–49 years old: 0–2.5 ng/ml 50–59 years old: 0–3.5 ng/ml 60–69 years old: 0–4.5 ng/ml 70–79 years old: 0–6.5 ng/ml	Account for normal increase in PSA that occurs with advancing age	Age ranges may improve specificity and positive predictive value of PSA testing; however, they also may decrease sensitivity for older men with increased acceptable PSA.
Race-specific PSA ranges	40–49 years old: 0–2, African Americans; 0–2.5, whites 50–59 years old: 0–4, African Americans; 0–3.5, whites 60–69 years old: 0–4.5, African Americans; 0–3.5, whites 70–79 years old: 0–5.5, African Americans; 0–3.5, whites	Accounts for racial differences in PSA values (possibly representing differences in prostate size), with increased PSA values commonly found among African Americans, adjusted for age, clinical stage, and histology	Utilization of race-specific ranges has not been associated with improved outcomes and is not currently recommended.
Human glandular kallikrein 2 (hK2)	Not established	Similar in structure to PSA; may be more specific to malignancy than benign prostate conditions.	Serum hK2 levels may correlate with prostate cancer.

Note. Based on information from Harris & Lohr, 2002; Loeb & Catalona, 2007; Roddam et al., 2005; Turner, 2007.

greatly assists in patient and provider decision making about PSA results and indications for biopsy. Given normal fluctuations of PSA levels in healthy men, often a second confirmatory PSA test is performed before proceeding to biopsy.

Increased prostate screening practices have resulted in the downward migration of stage at diagnosis and, therefore, greater likelihood of organ-confined disease. However, although "normal" PSA values do not exclude the possibility of cancer, the significance of intermediate PSA values (4–10 ng/ml) complicates the matter, as approximately 75% of these men will have a negative prostate biopsy (Spurgeon et al., 2007). In the presence of a normal DRE, the positive predictive value of an intermediate PSA level is approximately 25% (Crawford, Leewansangtong, Goktas, Holthaus, & Baier, 1999). Diagnostic activities in those with false-positive screening results (including prostate biopsy) contribute to significant anxiety, cancer-related worry, and short-term impact on sexual function (Katz et al., 2007). Therefore, this impact should be considered and anticipatory counseling provided for patients as they go through this process.

Serum PSA levels, DRE findings, and patient history are considered carefully to determine an estimate of the likelihood that prostate cancer is present. If these findings raise the suspicion of a potential prostate cancer, then prostate biopsy is the gold standard to confirm tissue diagnosis. The prostate biopsy can yield a great deal of information, including information about the histology, volume of glandular involvement with prostate cancer, and Gleason score (GS). Biopsy of the prostate base and seminal vesicles also may provide information about extension of prostate cancer beyond the prostate capsule. Details regarding the biopsy procedure are discussed later in this chapter.

Determining whether prostate cancer is organ confined or the disease extends beyond the prostate capsule is extremely important in making treatment recommendations, particularly for surgical resection. Therefore, depending on the risk of extraprostatic disease, further investigation may be required. Staging studies are selected to evaluate the presence of local invasion (extracapsular extension or seminal vesicle invasion), regional lymph node involvement, and metastatic disease. Risk-analysis nomograms have been investigated to assist in estimating the risk of nonlocalized disease; however, clinicians have simplified the stratification by designating three dominant risk groups based on the information noted earlier (American Urological Association, 2007; NCCN, 2007; Roach, Weinberg, Sandler, & Thompson, 2007).

- *Low risk:* PSA level ≤ 10 ng/ml, GS ≤ 6, and clinical stage T1–T2a
- *Intermediate risk:* PSA level = 10–20 ng/ml, or GS = 7, or clinical stage T2b (some T2c)
- *High risk:* PSA level > 20 ng/ml, or GS ≥ 8, or clinical stage T2c or T3a.

These risk groups are used for determining the need for further staging work-up as well as for treatment selection

purposes. Volume of prostate cancer involvement of sampled biopsy cores also has been identified as a potential prognostic indicator, with greater than five involved cores or greater than 50% sampled core tissue involvement being associated with greater risk of recurrent disease. Although this currently is not specifically included in risk or staging criteria, as further data emerge, it may be more formally incorporated in the future.

Staging

The Jewett staging system for prostate cancer was first introduced in 1975. This stratifies disease extent from A to D (stage A representing clinically undetectable disease, and stage D representing metastatic disease). The American Joint Committee on Cancer (AJCC)/International Union Against Cancer staging system for prostate cancer largely supplanted the Jewett staging system in 1997. The AJCC staging criteria were updated in 2002. Although induction PSA value and GS have yet to be included in the AJCC staging criteria, these parameters are considered (risk grouping) along with the staging information in determining treatment recommendations.

The purposes of the staging system are to provide a standardized way of describing tumor involvement for comparison of larger groups of patient outcomes and to stratify risk of cancer recurrence and survival. The current AJCC staging criteria are based on tumor size (T), lymph node status (N), and presence of metastasis (M) (Roach et al., 2007), each of which is categorized and then grouped to determine the overall disease stage (see Figure 2-2). *Clinical staging* (cTNM) is based on examination, as well as laboratory and radiographic information, whereas *pathologic staging* (pTNM) is determined after surgical removal of the tumor (prostatectomy with or without pelvic nodal dissection). Clinical staging is not as reliable, and a high percentage of patients with prostate cancer are "upstaged" following surgical excision and nodal dissection (Jager et al., 2000). This largely anatomically focused system does not yet adequately reflect the biochemical significance of disease risk, so other parameters often are considered to determine the overall risk grouping. Pretreatment PSA level is thought to be the most important predictor of biochemical recurrence following radiation and, along with the GS, also is associated with increased mortality risk (Roach et al.).

Nonpalpable prostate cancers are staged as T1 tumors (T1a or T1b if incidentally found on pathologic review after surgery for benign reasons, and T1c if identified as a result of an abnormal screening PSA value). For these incidental prostate cancers, the risk of ultimate progression and mortality seems to be most associated with high-grade disease (high GS) and high-volume disease (diffuse disease involving a significant percentage of sampled tissue) (Ekman, Adolfsson, & Gronberg, 1999). T2 tumors are either clinically palpable or visible on transrectal ultrasound (TRUS) but are confined to the prostate. T3 tumors are localized but extend through

Figure 2-2. American Joint Committee on Cancer and Jewett Staging

TNM definitions

Primary tumor (T)
- TX: Primary tumor cannot be assessed
- T0: No evidence of primary tumor
- T1: Clinically inapparent tumor not palpable nor visible by imaging
  - T1a: Tumor incidental histologic finding in 5% or less of tissue resected
  - T1b: Tumor incidental histologic finding in more than 5% of tissue resected
  - T1c: Tumor identified by needle biopsy (e.g., because of elevated prostate-specific antigen)
- T2: Tumor confined within prostate*
  - T2a: Tumor involves 50% or less of one lobe
  - T2b: Tumor involves more than 50% of one lobe but not both lobes
  - T2c: Tumor involves both lobes
- T3: Tumor extends through the prostate capsule**
  - T3a: Extracapsular extension (unilateral or bilateral)
  - T3b: Tumor invades seminal vesicle(s)
- T4: Tumor is fixed or invades adjacent structures other than seminal vesicles: bladder neck, external sphincter, rectum, levator muscles, and/or pelvic wall

*Note: Tumor that is found in one or both lobes by needle biopsy but is not palpable or reliably visible by imaging is classified as T1c.
**Note: Invasion into the prostatic apex or into (but not beyond) the prostatic capsule is classified as T2 not T3.

Regional lymph nodes (N)
Regional lymph nodes are the nodes of the true pelvis, which essentially are the pelvic nodes below the bifurcation of the common iliac arteries. They include the following groups (laterality does not affect the N classification): pelvic (not otherwise specified [NOS]), hypogastric, obturator, iliac (i.e., internal, external, or NOS), and sacral (lateral, presacral, promontory [e.g., Gerota], or NOS). Distant lymph nodes are outside the confines of the true pelvis. They can be imaged using ultrasound, CT, MRI, or lymphangiography and include: aortic (para-aortic, periaortic, or lumbar), common iliac, inguinal (deep), superficial inguinal (femoral), supraclavicular, cervical, scalene, and retroperitoneal (NOS) nodes. Although enlarged lymph nodes can occasionally be visualized, because of a stage migration associated with PSA screening, very few patients will be found to have nodal disease, so false-positive and false-negative results are common when imaging tests are employed. In lieu of imaging, risk tables are generally used to determine individual patient risk of nodal involvement. Involvement of distant lymph nodes is classified as M1a.
- NX: Regional lymph nodes were not assessed
- N0: No regional lymph node metastasis
- N1: Metastasis in regional lymph node(s)

Distant metastasis (M)*
- MX: Distant metastasis cannot be assessed (not evaluated by any modality)
- M0: No distant metastasis
- M1: Distant metastasis
  - M1a: Nonregional lymph node(s)
  - M1b: Bone(s)
  - M1c: Other site(s) with or without bone disease

*Note: When more than one site of metastasis is present, the most advanced category (pM1c) is used.

Histopathologic grade (G)
- GX: Grade cannot be assessed
- G1: Well-differentiated (slight anaplasia) (Gleason score of 2–4)
- G2: Moderately differentiated (moderate anaplasia) (Gleason score of 5–6)
- G3–4: Poorly differentiated or undifferentiated (marked anaplasia) (Gleason score of 7–10)

American Joint Committee on Cancer stage groupings
Stage I
- T1a, N0, M0, G1

Stage II
- T1a, N0, M0, G2–4
- T1b, N0, M0, any G
- T1c, N0, M0, any G
- T1, N0, M0, any G
- T2, N0, M0, any G

Stage III
- T3, N0, M0, any G

Stage IV
- T4, N0, M0, any G
- Any T, N1, M0, any G
- Any T, any N, M1, any G

(Continued on next page)

Figure 2-2. American Joint Committee on Cancer and Jewett Staging *(Continued)*

Jewett Staging System

Stage A

Stage A is clinically undetectable tumor confined to the prostate gland and is an incidental finding at prostatic surgery.
- Substage A1: well-differentiated with focal involvement and usually left untreated
- Substage A2: moderately or poorly differentiated or involves multiple foci in the gland

Stage B

Stage B is tumor confined to the prostate gland.
- Substage B0: nonpalpable and PSA-detected
- Substage B1: single nodule in one lobe of the prostate
- Substage B2: more extensive involvement of one lobe or involvement of both lobes

Stage C

Stage C is tumor clinically localized to the periprostatic area but extending through the prostatic capsule; seminal vesicles may be involved.
- Substage C1: clinical extracapsular extension
- Substage C2: extracapsular tumor producing bladder outlet or ureteral obstruction

Stage D

Stage D is metastatic disease.
- Substage D0: clinically localized disease (prostate only) but persistently elevated enzymatic serum acid phosphatase titers
- Substage D1: regional lymph nodes only
- Substage D2: distant lymph nodes and metastases to bone or visceral organs
- Substage D3: D2 prostate cancer patients who relapsed after adequate endocrine therapy

Note. From *Prostate Cancer Treatment (PDQ®): Stage Information,* by the National Cancer Institute, 2008. Retrieved March 20, 2008, from http://www.cancer.gov/cancertopics/pdq/treatment/prostate/HealthProfessional/page4

---

the prostate capsule or involve one or both of the seminal vesicles. Penetration through the prostatic capsule typically is a relatively late event and may indicate a more aggressive tumor type with higher risk of local recurrence and metastatic disease.

Definitive therapy with curative intent (surgery, brachytherapy, external beam radiation) generally is offered to patients with evidence of localized disease and life expectancy of greater than 10 years (Bott et al., 2007). Therefore, accurate staging, as well as appraisal of the pathologic features of the tumor and patients' overall health condition, is essential in making appropriate treatment recommendations. Given the importance of prostate cancer staging, several guidelines exist to enhance provider consistency and appropriate selection of staging studies. NCCN, the American Urological Association, and ACR have all published guidelines for prostate cancer diagnosis, staging, and treatment over the past 10 years, and adherence to the guidelines has largely resulted in more appropriate intervention selection (Abraham et al., 2007).

Staging Guidelines

American College of Radiology

ACR first published guidelines for pretreatment staging of localized prostate cancer in 2003, which were updated in 2005. The goal of the guidelines is to assist clinicians in determining the appropriate utilization of available imaging tests to stage prostate cancer based on risk criteria. T stage, GS, pretreatment PSA level, and volume of biopsy core disease involvement is grouped, and common imaging modalities are weighted from least to most appropriate for each grouping.

National Comprehensive Cancer Network

Whereas the ACR guidelines aim to guide selection of imaging to improve appropriate utilization and test selection, the NCCN guidelines for prostate cancer diagnosis and staging provide an algorithm guiding work-up to improve diagnostic consistency and accuracy of staging (see Figure 2-3). The guidelines provide evidence-based criteria for obtaining further diagnostic studies based on risk stratification.

Clinical Examination

Obtaining a clinical history and general physical exam is always an important aspect of a thorough evaluation. In the setting of a newly diagnosed patient with prostate cancer, the evaluation is conducted to determine the extent of localized disease, to evaluate symptoms related to the disease (and symptoms of potential metastatic disease, such as bone pain), and also to determine the patients' overall health status and life expectancy. Life expectancy (rather than specific age) is a major treatment decision factor (American Urological Association, 2007). The likelihood of prostate-related morbidity and mortality is greater for those with long life expectancies than for those with significant comorbidities and relatively

---

Figure 2-3. National Comprehensive Cancer Network Prostate Cancer Diagnosis and Staging Guidelines

Initial studies:
- Digital rectal exam
- Prostate-specific antigen (PSA)
- Biopsy with Gleason score (GS) determination

If life expectancy estimated > 5 years, symptomatic, OR high risk features (T3-4 disease or GS ≥ 8) and/or symptomatic:
- Pelvic computed tomography/magnetic resonance imaging
  - T3–T4
  - T1–T2 AND > 20% estimated risk of lymph node involvement
- Bone scan
  - Clinical symptoms
  - T3–T4 stage
  - T1–T2 stage AND PSA > 20, OR GS > 8

Note. Based on information from National Comprehensive Cancer Network, 2008.

---

shorter life expectancy (less than 10 years) (American Urological Association). However, valid concern exists that no reliable method is currently available for accurately determining life expectancy (McCloskey & Kuettel, 2007).

DRE is integral to prostate cancer screening and is essential in the diagnostic and staging process for prostate cancer. The surface of the small walnut-shaped gland may be readily evaluated by palpation of the rectal wall. The region of the prostate adjacent to the rectal wall is the most common site for tumors to occur (American Urological Association, 2007). Although cancer occurring in the posterior and lateral aspects of the prostate can be identified, approximately 25%–35% of prostate cancers occur in other parts of the gland (i.e., anteriorly) and are not palpable. Presence of induration (firmness), asymmetry, or any palpable nodules should be noted and prompt further evaluation (biopsy), even in the presence of low serum PSA levels. The volume of disease, as well as unilateral, bilateral, or multifocal disease involvement, also should be noted. The seminal vesicles can be examined for clinical evidence of disease spread, although DRE is relatively insensitive in determining the presence of extracapsular invasion. DRE findings must be interpreted with caution. Often other imaging studies will be required, as DRE frequently underestimates T staging. Approximately 50% of palpable prostate nodules result in the finding of cancer on biopsy. A serum PSA value should be obtained prior to performing the DRE, as serum PSA levels may be elevated in the first few hours after the exam, but the increase is relatively small (Loeb & Catalona, 2007).

Laboratory Evaluation

The primary laboratory study used in the diagnosis and staging of prostate cancer is the serum PSA value (as described previously in this chapter). However, prostatic acid phosphatase (PAP) also has been used to evaluate prostate cancer. Prostatic epithelial cells secrete PAP, which may be elevated in extracapsular disease as well as following prostate manipulation or because of prostatitis. As a result of increased PSA screening and earlier diagnosis of disease, PAP measurements add little information to clinical staging (Canto, Shariat, & Slawin, 2003). A complete blood count and chemistry panel also may be helpful in detecting other consequences related to more advanced prostate cancer (such as anemia, renal function, or possible elevated alkaline phosphatase, potentially indicating osseous metastasis). Additionally, prothrombin time, international normalized ratio (INR), and partial thromboplastin time should be obtained prior to surgical prostatectomy but are not routinely necessary prior to prostate biopsy.

Many other molecular markers of prostate cancer are under investigation. An investigational reverse transcriptase polymerase chain reaction test for serum PSA mRNA may accurately detect circulating PSA-producing cells; however, this is not predictive for tumor stage or disease volume; therefore, the clinical utility of this method is uncertain.

Radiographic Evaluation

Several imaging modalities are available for more accurate clinical staging of newly diagnosed prostate cancer, but precise indications for and sensitivity and specificity of many conventional radiographic methods remain controversial (Hricak, Choyke, Eberhardt, Leibel, & Scardino, 2007). Evidence-based guidelines are available to help to ensure that judicious use of imaging is balanced with the need for complete staging work-up. More appropriate utilization of imaging, as well as downward stage migration because of PSA screening, has led to progressive decline in image testing overall with the greatest decline in imaging occurring in low-risk-group patients (Cooperberg, Lubeck, Grossfeld, Mehta, & Carroll, 2002). As always, consideration of what imaging is appropriate should be based on what questions need to be answered in light of how it will change the course of clinical care.

Radionuclide Bone Scan

Although a radionuclide bone scan serves no role in the diagnosis and staging of localized prostate cancer, it is useful in detecting metastatic osseous involvement. The sensitivity of bone scans for detecting bone metastasis is quite good, particularly for osteoblastic lesions, which demonstrate increased radiotracer uptake in comparison to uninvolved bone (Hricak et al., 2007). Bone scans often demonstrate evidence of bone involvement prior to the development of clinical symptoms (such as bone pain) and appear to be more sensitive than conventional radiographs for metastatic osseous detection (Palmer, Henrikson, McKusick, Strauss, & Hochberg, 1988).

A staging bone scan for men with a PSA level of greater than 20 ng/ml to rule out distant disease before embarking on curative therapy is considered standard of care. Increased PSA values correlate with the likelihood of a positive bone scan result. Positive bone scans with low PSA levels (less than 8 ng/ml) are uncommon (Oesterling, Martin, Bergstralh, & Lowe, 1993), whereas a 10% incidence of positive bone scan findings occurs when PSA levels are 10–50 ng/ml, which increases to 50% risk when the PSA value is greater than 50 ng/ml (Hricak et al., 2007). Staging bone scans therefore are not considered necessary for early-stage tumors (T1 and T2) with a low serum PSA level (less than 10 ng/ml) and a GS of less than 6.

Computed Tomography

Abdominal and pelvic computed tomography (CT) scanning frequently is considered in the staging work-up for prostate cancer but often results in negative findings. It may be more useful in the evaluation of advanced disease, and its use in primary staging of early prostate cancer (apart from treatment planning) perhaps is limited. Pelvic adenopathy may be identified but is not common in early-stage prostate cancer, and microscopic nodal involvement is not detectable on CT. CT scans do not clearly visualize intraprostatic anatomy and have poor sensitivity for extraprostatic extension and seminal vesicle invasion and therefore do not adequately ensure localized disease (Hricak et al., 2007). In men with greater risk of lymph node involvement (i.e., advanced clinical stage, high PSA value, high GS), CT scanning should be performed, and men who anticipate undergoing external beam radiotherapy should have a CT scan for treatment planning purposes.

Magnetic Resonance Imaging

Optimal prostate imaging with magnetic resonance imaging (MRI) requires use of an endorectal coil with a pelvic phased-array coil on a mid- to high-field-strength magnet (Hricak et al., 2007). During the exam, a rectal probe is placed for magnetic resonance (MR) visualization of the prostate gland and associated structures. Imaging may be delayed at least three weeks, and often six to eight weeks, after prostate biopsy to ensure that accuracy of interpretation is not hampered by subsequent hemorrhage. Currently, endorectal coil MRI (ER-MRI) is the method of choice for detecting extraprostatic extension and seminal vesicle invasion (see Figure 2-4). This may be helpful in distinguishing those with prostate-confined disease from those with extracapsular disease when making treatment decisions, such as surgery.

MRI has limited value in the detection of prostate cancer, but it may be considered in cases of suspected prostate cancer where TRUS and biopsy findings are negative (Hricak et al., 2007). Optimal use of ER-MRI in prostate cancer staging has not clearly been defined, and wide variations exist in practice among institutions. Routine preoperative use of staging ER-MRI is somewhat controversial, as it is unclear

Figure 2-4. Endorectal Coil Magnetic Resonance Imaging of the Prostate

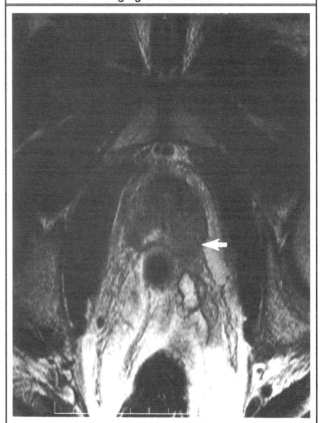

There is a subtle breach in the integrity of the prostatic capsule at the left base, mid-gland, suggesting evidence of extracapsular extension.

Note. Figure courtesy of Virginia Mason Medical Center, Seattle, WA. Used with permission.

whether it commonly adds to clinical decision making (Jager et al., 2000).

MRI also may be used for specific evaluation of osseous metastasis, as it has high sensitivity and specificity for metastatic bone lesions. It is somewhat impractical for generalized skeletal survey, therefore making radionuclide bone scan the test of choice for this purpose.

MR spectroscopic (MR-S) imaging increases the sensitivity of MRI (particularly for transition zone lesions) and adds information about metabolic characteristics of the tumor (Hricak et al., 2007; Zakian et al., 2003). MR-S displays relative variations in metabolite concentrations (citrate, creatine, and choline when used for prostate cancer detection) within a small area. Differences in the biology of normal prostate tissue, which secretes citrate, and prostate cancer, which is associated with increased choline concentrations resulting from increased proliferative activity, are visually represented. Therefore, beyond providing anatomic characteristics, MR-S also provides biologic information about the tumor, and correlation of MR-S findings with tumor aggressiveness and GS has been suggested (Zakian et al., 2005). In the future, MR-S may play a role in guiding high-dose intraprostatic radiation treatment to areas of concern.

ProstaScint Scan

The ProstaScint® (capromab pendetide) scan (Cytogen Corp.) utilizes indium-111 capromab pendetide, a radiolabeled monoclonal antibody specific to prostate-specific membrane antigen (PSMA), which is highly expressed in malignant prostate cells, to identify soft tissue and intra- and extraprostatic prostate cancer (Taneja, 2004). This may be useful during initial staging to determine whether extraprostatic, nodal, or other metastatic soft tissue involvement is present that may be difficult to identify with other imaging (such as CT or MRI). Initially, the sensitivity of the ProstaScint technique was suboptimal (particularly in patients with low-volume disease); however, over the past several years, improvement in single photon emission CT imaging technology, CT fusion capability, and greater interpretation experience has led to renewed interest in the test's clinical utility. Given the favorable negative predictive value of the ProstaScint scan, its use in intermediate- to high-risk patients may be particularly helpful in selecting those who are appropriate for potentially curative therapy (Taneja). Furthermore, in men with biochemical relapse following definitive treatment, the ProstaScint scan may help to distinguish those with isolated prostate or prostate bed recurrence (i.e., who would benefit from local therapy) from those with distant metastatic disease. The impact of effect on long-term outcomes in this setting has been controversial, however (Nagda et al., 2007). One retrospective study of 44 men undergoing salvage radiotherapy for biochemical relapse following prostatectomy found that although ProstaScint imaging predicted improved survival for those patients with negative pretreatment scans, this finding was not independent of pre-radiation PSA values, thus making the added benefit of the test unclear (Proano, Sodee, Resnick, & Einstein, 2006). Molecular imaging has the advantage of better visualizing microscopic disease than other conventional imaging techniques, which may be of benefit for selected patients although routine clinical use is not yet supported.

Transrectal Ultrasound

TRUS often is performed in the evaluation of prostate cancer. It may assist in the evaluation and characterization of abnormalities found on DRE and to estimate the size of the prostate (important for treatment planning); however, its primary utility is to aid in localization during prostate biopsy. TRUS guidance for brachytherapy seed placement and cryotherapy of the prostate also is used. During TRUS, the patient is placed in decubitus position, and a rectally inserted ultrasound probe is used to evaluate the prostate and seminal vesicles (Hricak et al., 2007). Malignant nodules often appear hypoechoic on ultrasound, although hyperechoic or isoechoic lesions may also rarely represent cancer (Shinohara, Wheeler, & Scardino, 1989).

The sensitivity of TRUS in detecting seminal vesicle invasion and extracapsular extension has declined somewhat because of downward stage migration over the past several years, as tumors are smaller and incidence of seminal vesicle invasion and extracapsular spread is less common (Hricak et al., 2007). The addition of color duplex Doppler and color power Doppler ultrasound (to detect cancer in hypervascular areas) may slightly improve ultrasound sensitivity and specificity (Halpern et al., 2002).

Prostate Biopsy

Prostate biopsy is a relatively simple office procedure, commonly performed without sedation or analgesia. Topical anesthetic or local infiltration of an anesthetic into the periprostatic tissue may be performed, but for many, the placement of the ultrasound probe may be equal to or more uncomfortable than the actual needle biopsy (Luscombe & Cooke, 2004). Hematuria, hematospermia, rectal bleeding, fever, and urinary retention have occurred following transrectal prostate biopsy, and some symptoms may occur for up to a week following biopsy (Raaijmakers, Kirkels, Roobol, Wildhagen, & Schrder, 2002). Men should receive routine counseling about the potential for such side effects. Patients should avoid anticoagulants (including aspirin and nonsteroidal anti-inflammatory drugs) 10 days prior to biopsy. Patients also require preparation with an enema and antibiotic administration before the biopsy and should expect to receive an antibiotic prescription on discharge after the procedure (Hricak et al., 2007).

Prostate cancer often is a multifocal disease, commonly presenting with multiple microscopic areas of involvement within the prostate. A greater number of cores sampled during biopsy increases the likelihood of disease detection, with an average of 10–12 cores currently recommended (Takenaka et al., 2006). However, some physicians utilize a prostate biopsy procedure that includes the use of two consecutive sets of sextant biopsies, which may yield as many as 8–32 core biopsy samples (Carter, DeMarzo, & Lilja, 2004). Prostate cancers occur most frequently in the posterior region of the prostate gland; therefore, biopsies generally are taken from the medial and lateral aspects of the apex, mid-gland, and base on both sides of the gland in the peripheral zone (Thompson & Ankerst, 2007). Additional biopsies also are taken of any abnormal areas detected by DRE or TRUS findings, including the seminal vesicles if extraprostatic extension at the base of the gland is suspected (Hricak et al., 2007). Anterior prostate sampling (transitional zone) generally is not performed unless previous biopsies have not elicited a diagnosis in those suspected of having prostate cancer or if imaging suggests presence of an anterior lesion (Hricak et al.). The pathologist inspects the sampled cores (generally

1–1.5 cm in length and 0.1 cm in diameter) microscopically to determine tumor histology, volume of tumor involvement, and differentiation (GS).

It has been suggested that prostate biopsy in certain specific selected populations may not add significantly to treatment decisions. A study of 205 men older than age 80 determined that PSA testing alone was a good predictor of positive biopsy (PSA level ≥ 30 ng/ml correlated with 96% occurrence of positive prostate biopsy) (Bott et al., 2007). For those in whom androgen suppression therapy alone would be considered, obtaining a prostate biopsy did not alter treatment recommendations. Very healthy 80-year-old men with a greater than 10-year life expectancy who may consider radiation would benefit from information gained from prostate biopsy; however, for a carefully selected population, forgoing prostate biopsy may be safely considered. Most clinicians, however, would be reluctant to actively treat a patient in the absence of a positive biopsy result.

Histopathology

Pathologic review of the prostate tissue is evaluated to determine the tissue type, tumor grade, and presence of any significant risk factors. Adenocarcinoma is the most common histopathologic type of prostate cancer, accounting for approximately 95% of diagnoses. Transitional cell carcinoma, basal cell carcinoma, lymphoma, stromal sarcoma, small cell tumors, and carcinoid (neuroendocrine) tumors also may occur in the prostate but are much less common.

Prostatic intraepithelial neoplasia (PIN) is a benign pathologic finding with little clinical significance; however, high-grade PIN may be a precursor lesion for cancer development and is therefore commonly identified when present in the biopsy report.

Although still somewhat limited, the GS is the best predictor of the biologic aggressiveness of prostate tumors. Differentiation patterns of the cancer cells are graded with a score of one to five (with one being well differentiated, and five representing undifferentiated cancer cells) (see Figure 2-5). The GS represents the sum of both the dominant and less dominant architectural growth differentiation patterns; therefore, a total score of 10 is possible, with a higher score indicating greater risk of treatment failure.

The pathology report also may identify other indicators of tumor aggressiveness, such as periprostatic invasion. Extracapsular extension is a poor prognostic finding, indicative of more aggressive tumor biology. Prostate cancer occurring in the peripheral zone is more likely to extend into the ejaculatory ducts and seminal vesicles, and these areas are not uncommonly included in the biopsy if suspicion of invasion is present. Perineural or perivascular invasion, if present, also raises concern for greater risk of treatment failure.

Unlike some other cancer sites (such as breast cancer), limited information about molecular markers is available to guide treatment. This is partly because of the comparative lack of available prostate tissue for research purposes, as unfixed/

Figure 2-5. Gleason Grading System

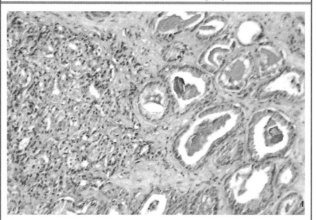

Histological slide (hematoxylin and eosin [H & E] stain at x 300) showing prostate cancer. On the right is a somewhat normal Gleason value of 3 (out of 5) with moderately differentiated cancer. On the left is less normal tissue with a Gleason value of 4 (out of 5) that is highly undifferentiated. The Gleason score is the sum of the two worst areas of the histological slide.

Note. Image created by Otis Brawley; used courtesy of the National Cancer Institute.

frozen prostate tissue is only rarely collected from patients with prostate cancer (Schlomm, Erbersdobler, Mirlacher, & Sauter, 2007). Several prognostic and predictive markers are under investigation for their potential role in appropriate treatment selection in prostate cancer (see Table 2-2).

Conclusion

The primary aim of the staging evaluation for a newly diagnosed patient with prostate cancer is to distinguish metastatic from organ-confined disease. This has significant treatment implications and is essential in making appropriate therapeutic recommendations. In addition to anatomic staging, biologic activity also is considered in risk stratification. Although not formally included in staging criteria, oncologists have "spoken with their feet" by agreeing on the correlating risk levels of PSA values and GS and using these parameters to guide therapy. An array of imaging modalities are available, and appropriate selection is based on stage, likelihood of a positive outcome, and how the results will affect treatment options. As technology continues to become more sophisticated, more sensitive laboratory, pathologic, and radiographic modalities will improve clinicians' ability to differentiate the "clinically insignificant" from the biologically aggressive prostate cancers. Until then, each case must be carefully evaluated within the context of risks and likelihoods, and patients should be fully informed of the expected benefits and limitations of screening, staging, and treatment.

Table 2-2. Potential Prognostic or Predictive Molecular Markers in Prostate Cancer	
Marker	**Role**
p53	Tumor suppressor gene may be associated with worse outcomes, possible predictor of radiation resistance
Bcl-2	Apoptosis-inhibiting protein, may be associated with worse prognosis
Ki67 labeling index	Measure of cellular proliferation activity, related to Gleason score, and may correlate with prognostic outcomes or risk of recurrence
Androgen receptor/prostate-specific antigen (PSA)	Decreased tumor expression of PSA and androgen receptor expression have been associated with worse prognosis.
E-cadherin	Adhesion molecules; decreased expression of these alpha/beta-catenin molecules has been associated with higher Gleason score.
P27^{Kip1}	Negative regulator of cell proliferation; decreased expression in prostate tumors has been associated with higher T stage/Gleason score and worse prognosis (but also has been observed in benign prostate hyperplastic tissue).
Neuroendocrine differentiation	May predict poor response to radiation and antiandrogen therapy; has poor correlation with prognostic outcomes
Prostate-specific membrane antigen	Overexpressed on membranes of most prostate tumor cells; may correlate with poor prognosis; may be suitable target for drug therapy
HER2	HER2 amplification has been observed in some prostate cancers; however, trastuzumab did not demonstrate clinical impact—low-level HER2 expression may be predictive of worse prognosis.
Epidermal growth factor receptor (EGFR)	High EGFR may be predictive of worse prognosis; role for anti-EGFR drugs in prostate cancer is being evaluated.

Note. Based on information from Schlomm et al., 2007; Scott et al., 2003.

References

Abraham, N., Wan, F., Montagnet, C., Wong, Y.N., & Armstrong, K. (2007). Decrease in racial disparities in the staging evaluation for prostate cancer after publication of staging guidelines. *Journal of Urology, 178*(1), 82–87.

American Urological Association. (2007). *Prostate cancer: Guideline for the management of clinically localized prostate cancer: 2007 update.* Linthicum, MD: American Urological Association Education and Research.

Bostwick, D.G., Burke, H.B., Djakiew, D., Euling, S., Ho, S.M., Landolph, J., et al. (2004). Human prostate cancer risk factors. *Cancer, 101*(Suppl. 10), 2371–2490.

Bott, S., Foley, C.L., Bull, M.D., Reddy, C.C., Freeman, A., Montgomery, B.S., et al. (2007). Are prostatic biopsies necessary in men aged ≥ 80 years? *BJU International, 99*(2), 335–338.

Canto, E.L., Shariat, S.F., & Slawin, K.M. (2003). Biochemical staging of prostate cancer. *Urologic Clinics of North America, 30*(2), 263–277.

Carter, H.B., DeMarzo, A., & Lilja, H. (2004). Detection, diagnosis, and prognosis of prostate cancer. In *Report to the nation on prostate cancer 2004.* Retrieved February 26, 2008, from http://www.medscape.com/viewprogram/3440

Cooperberg, M.R., Lubeck, D.P., Grossfeld, G.D., Mehta, S.S., & Carroll, P.R. (2002). Contemporary trends in imaging test utilization in prostate cancer staging: Data from the Cancer of the Prostate Strategic Urologic Research Endeavor. *Journal of Urology, 168*(2), 491–495.

Crawford, E.D., Leewansangtong, S., Goktas, S., Holthaus, K., & Baier, M. (1999). Efficiency of prostate-specific antigen and digital rectal examination in screening, using 4.0 ng/ml and age-specific reference range as a cutoff for abnormal values. *Prostate, 38*(4), 296–302.

Ekman, P., Adolfsson, J., & Gronberg, H. (1999). The natural history of prostate cancer. In A.V. Kaisary, G.P. Murphy, L. Denis, & K. Griffiths (Eds.), *Textbook of prostate cancer: Pathology, diagnosis and treatment* (pp. 1–16). Malden, MA: Blackwell Science.

Halpern, E.J., Frauscher, F., Strup, S.E., Nazarian, L.N., O'Kane, P., & Gomella, L.G. (2002). Prostate: High-frequency Doppler US imaging for cancer detection. *Radiology, 225*(1), 71–77.

Harris, R., & Lohr, K.N. (2002). Screening for prostate cancer: An update of the evidence. *Annals of Internal Medicine, 137*(11), 917–929.

Hricak, H., Choyke, P.L., Eberhardt, S.C., Leibel, S.A., & Scardino, P.T. (2007). Imaging prostate cancer: Multidisciplinary perspective. *Radiology, 243*(1), 28–53.

Jager, G.J., Severens, J.L., Thornbury, J.R., de La Rosette, J.J., Ruijs, S.H., & Barentsz, J.O. (2000). Prostate cancer staging: Should MR imaging be used? A decision analytic approach. *Radiology, 215*(2), 445–451.

Jemal, A., Siegel, R., Ward, E., Hao, Y., Xu, J., Murray, T., et al. (2008). Cancer statistics, 2008. *CA: A Cancer Journal for Clinicians, 58*(2), 71–96.

Katz, D.A., Jarrard, D.F., McHorney, C.A., Hillis, S.L., Wieve, D.A., & Fryback, D.G. (2007). Health perceptions in patients who undergo screening and workup for prostate cancer. *Urology, 69*(2), 215–220.

Loeb, S., & Catalona, W.J. (2007). Prostate-specific antigen in clinical practice. *Cancer Letters, 249*(1), 30–39.

Luscombe, C.J., & Cooke, P.W. (2004). Pain during prostate biopsy. *Lancet, 363*(9424), 1840–1841.

McCloskey, S.A., & Kuettel, M.R. (2007). Counterpoint: Prostate cancer life expectancy can not be accurately predicted from currently available tools. *Journal of the National Comprehensive Cancer Network, 5*(7), 709–713.

Nagda, S.N., Mohideen, N., Lo, S.S., Khan, U., Dillehay, G., Wagner, R., et al. (2007). Long-term follow-up of ^{111}In-capromab pendetide (ProstaScint) scan as pretreatment assessment in patients who undergo salvage radiotherapy for rising prostate-specific antigen after radical prostatectomy for prostate cancer. *International Journal of Radiation Oncology, Biology, Physics, 67*(3), 834–840.

Nam, R.K., Toi, A., Klotz, L.H., Trachtenberg, J., Jewett, M., Appu, S., et al. (2007). Assessing individual risk for prostate cancer. *Journal of Clinical Oncology, 25*(24), 3582–3588.

National Comprehensive Cancer Network. (2007). *NCCN Clinical Practice Guidelines in Oncology™: Prostate cancer early detection* [v.2.2007]. Retrieved July 14, 2008, from http://www.nccn.org/professionals/physician_gls/PDF/prostate_detection.pdf

National Comprehensive Cancer Network. (2008). *NCCN Clinical Practice Guidelines in Oncology™: Prostate cancer* [v.1.2008]. Retrieved July 14, 2008, from http://www.nccn.org/professionals/physician_gls/PDF/prostate.pdf

Oesterling, J.E., Martin, S.K., Bergstralh, E.J., & Lowe, F.C. (1993). The use of prostate specific antigen in staging patients with newly diagnosed prostate cancer. *JAMA, 269*(1), 57–60.

Palmer, E., Henrikson, B., McKusick, K., Strauss, H.W., & Hochberg, F. (1988). Pain as an indicator of bone metastasis. *Acta Radiologica, 29*(4), 445–449.

Proano, J.M., Sodee, D.B., Resnick, M.I., & Einstein, D.B. (2006). The impact of a negative (111)indium-capromab pendetide scan before salvage radiotherapy. *Journal of Urology, 175*(5), 1668–1672.

Raaijmakers, R., Kirkels, W.J., Roobol, M.J., Wildhagen, M.F., & Schrder, F.H. (2002). Complication rates and risk factors of 5802 transrectal ultrasound-guided sextant biopsies of the prostate within a population-based screening program. *Urology, 60*(5), 826–830.

Roach, M., Weinberg, V., Sandler, H., & Thompson, I. (2007). Staging for prostate cancer: Time to incorporate pretreatment prostate-specific antigen and Gleason score? *Cancer, 109*(2), 213–220.

Roddam, A.W., Duffy, M.J., Hamdy, F.C., Ward, A.M., Patnick, J., Price, C.P., et al. (2005). Use of prostate-specific antigen (PSA) isoforms for the detection of prostate cancer in men with a PSA level of 2–10 ng/ml: systematic review and meta-analysis. *European Urology, 48*(3), 386–399.

Schlomm, T., Erbersdobler, A., Mirlacher, M., & Sauter, G. (2007). Molecular staging of prostate cancer in the year 2007. *World Journal of Urology, 25*(1), 19–30.

Scott, S.L., Earle, J.D., & Gumerlock, P.H. (2003). Functional p53 increases prostate cancer cell survival after exposure to fractionated doses of ionizing radiation. *Cancer Research, 63*(21), 7190–7196.

Shinohara, K., Wheeler, T.M., & Scardino, P.T. (1989). The appearance of prostate cancer on transrectal ultrasonography: Correlation of imaging and pathological exams. *Journal of Urology, 142*(1), 76–82.

Spurgeon, S., Mongoue-Tchokote, S., Collins, L., Priest, R., Hsieh, Y., Peters, L.M., et al. (2007). Assessment of prostate-specific antigen doubling time in prediction of prostate cancer on needle biopsy. *Urology, 69*(5), 931–935.

Takenaka, A., Hara, R., Hyodo, Y., Ishimura, T., Sakai, Y., Fujioka, H., et al. (2006). Transperineal extended biopsy improves the clinically significant prostate cancer detections rate: A comparative study of 6 and 12 biopsy cores. *International Journal of Urology, 13*(1), 10–14.

Taneja, S.S. (2004). ProstaScint® scan: Contemporary use in clinical practice. *Reviews in Urology, 6*(Suppl. 10), S19–S28.

Thompson, I.M., & Ankerst, D.P. (2007). Prostate-specific antigen in the early detection of prostate cancer. *Canadian Medical Association Journal, 176*(13), 1853–1858.

Thompson, I.M., Ankerst, D.P., Chi, C., Goodman, P.J., Tangen, C.M., Lucia, M.S., et al. (2006). Assessing prostate cancer risk: Results from the Prostate Cancer Prevention Trial. *Journal of the National Cancer Institute, 98*(8), 529–534.

Thompson, I.M., Pauler, D.K., Goodman, P.J., Tangen, C.M., Lucia, M.S., Parnes, H.L., et al. (2004). Prevalence of prostate cancer among men with a prostate-specific antigen level < or = 4.0 ng per milliliter. *New England Journal of Medicine, 350*(22), 2239–2246.

Turner, B. (2007). Diagnosis and treatment of patients with prostate cancer: The nurse's role. *Nursing Standard, 21*(39), 48–56.

Vickers, A.J., Ulmert, D., Serio, A.M., Bjork, T., Scardino, P.T., Eastham, J.A., et al. (2007). The predictive value of prostate cancer biomarkers depends on age and time to diagnosis: Towards a biologically-based screening strategy. *International Journal of Cancer, 121*(10), 2212–2217.

Zakian, K.L., Eberhardt, S., Hricak, H., Shukla-Dave, A., Kleinman, S., Muruganandham, M., et al. (2003). Transition zone prostate cancer: Metabolic characteristics at 1H MR spectroscopic imaging—initial results. *Radiology, 229*(1), 241–247.

Zakian, K.L., Sircar, K., Hricak, H., Chen, H.N., Shukla-Dave, A., Eberhardt, S., et al. (2005). Correlation of proton MR spectroscopic imaging with Gleason score based on step-section pathologic analysis after radical prostatectomy. *Radiology, 234*(3), 804–814.

CHAPTER 3

Prostate Cancer Screening, Risk, Prevention, and Prognosis

William P. Hogle, RN, MSN, OCN®

Introduction

Although it is fairly well known among healthcare professionals that prostate cancer is the most common noncutaneous malignancy among men in many parts of the Western world, the exact cause of the disease remains a mystery. A number of influential variables continue to be debated and researched as to their effect on the development and prevention of prostate cancer. The development of prostate-specific antigen (PSA)-based screening, initiated in 1989, has led to increased rates of early detection (McDavid, Lee, Fulton, Tonita, & Thompson, 2004) and has been a relatively effective measure of one's response to therapy. This chapter will discuss screening recommendations and controversies related to prostate cancer, examine the influence that risk factors have on the development of prostate cancer, and examine strategies used to prevent the disease. Furthermore, predictive models of disease outcomes will be examined to assist oncology nurses in educating patients regarding treatment options and quality-of-life concerns.

To Screen or Not to Screen

Screening for prostate cancer remains a controversial issue. Scientific data proving the effectiveness of PSA screening are still lacking with respect to the prevention of deaths from prostate cancer and whether it will outweigh the changes in quality of life experienced by men who have undergone treatment for the disease (Roobol, Grenabo, Schroder, & Hugosson, 2007). In 1984, the estimated incidence of prostate cancer was 5.1%, and by 1990, this number had risen to 60.6% (Jones et al., 1995). Between 1988 and 1995, a short-term rapid increase and subsequent decrease occurred in prostate cancer incidence rates (Jemal et al., 2008). From 1995 through 2004, incidence rates stabilized. These trends are believed to reflect changes in utilization of PSA testing (Espey et al., 2007; Jemal et al.).

Some clinicians advocate for screening of all men who reach a particular age, whereas others believe only those at high risk or those with multiple risk factors should undergo screening. In fact, some question the value of screening for men with less than a 10-year life expectancy or for those who are at high risk of dying from other comorbidities (Hoffman, Blume, & Gilliland, 1998; U.S. Preventive Services Task Force, 2002). Major organizations in favor of prostate cancer screening include the American Cancer Society (ACS), the American College of Radiology, the American Urological Association, the National Comprehensive Cancer Network (NCCN), and the Prostate Education Council. Organizations frequently sponsor prostate cancer screening programs, especially during the month of September, which is National Prostate Cancer Awareness Month. As a result, many men have taken part in such programs. Sirovich, Schwartz, and Woloshin (2003) estimated that approximately 75% of men older than age 50 have participated in prostate screening. See Table 3-1 for a summary of prostate cancer screening recommendations from selected organizations.

The current ACS guidelines for prostate cancer screening include annual digital rectal examination (DRE) and PSA testing in men older than age 50 with at least a 10-years life expectancy. Men at higher risk for disease (i.e., those of African descent or those with a first-degree relative with prostate cancer) should begin screening at age 45 (ACS, 2008).

Updated screening guidelines from NCCN include baseline DRE and PSA testing at age 40. If the PSA level is less than 0.6 ng/ml, the test should not be repeated until age 45. If the level remains the same at age 45, regular screening should not be started until age 50. If the initial PSA level is greater than 0.6 ng/ml or if the patient is at high risk, annual follow-up with repeat PSA testing and DRE should take place. If after one year the PSA level remains greater than 0.6 ng/ml, annual follow-up screening should continue. If the PSA value is less than 0.6 ng/ml after one year, screening should not be repeated until age 45. If at that time the level remains less than 0.6 ng/ml, screening should not be resumed until age 50 (NCCN, 2007).

Table 3-1. Summary of Prostate Cancer Screening Recommendations

Organization	Recommendation
American Academy of Family Physicians (2008)	Insufficient evidence exists on which to make a recommendation for or against screening for prostate cancer using prostate-specific antigen (PSA) testing or digital rectal examination (DRE).
American Cancer Society (2007)	Annual examination begins at age 50 for patients with at least a 10-year life expectancy. Men at higher risk (African Americans and those having first-degree relatives with prostate cancer) should begin testing at age 45. Information should be provided to all men about what is known and what is uncertain about the benefits and limitations of early detection and treatment of prostate cancer so that they can make informed decisions about testing.
American College of Physicians (1997)	Physicians should describe potential benefits and known harms of prostate cancer screening, diagnosis, and treatment; listen to the patient's concerns; and individualize the decision to screen.
American College of Preventive Medicine (Ferrini & Woolf, 1998)	Population screening with DRE and PSA testing is not recommended. Men aged 50 years or older with a life expectancy of more than 10 years should be given information about the potential benefits and harms of screening to allow them to make their own choices about screening.
American College of Radiology (Ferrini & Woolf, 1998)	Begin annual DRE and PSA screening at age 50; African American men and men with a positive family history of prostate cancer should have an annual PSA screening and DRE beginning at age 40.
American Medical Association (2001)	Both PSA testing and DRE should be offered annually, beginning at age 50, to men who have at least a 10-year life expectancy and to younger men who are at high risk.
Agency for Healthcare Research and Quality (U.S. Preventive Services Task Force, 2008)	Insufficient evidence exists on which to assess the balance of benefits and harms of prostate cancer screening in men younger than age 75 years. In addition, screening for prostate cancer in men age 73 years or older is not recommended.

Note. From "Reducing Prostate Cancer Morbidity and Mortality in African American Men: Issues and Challenges," by R.A. Jones, S.M. Underwood, and B.M. Rivers, 2007, *Clinical Journal of Oncology Nursing, 11*(6), p. 868. Copyright 2007 by the Oncology Nursing Society. Adapted with permission. Also based on information from U.S. Preventive Services Task Force, 2008.

In 1993, the National Cancer Institute (NCI) opened the Prostate, Lung, Colorectal, and Ovarian Cancer Screening Trial, a randomized trial in which 148,000 men and women ages 55–74 were enrolled and evaluated for cancer at periodic intervals (Andriole et al., 2005). The purposes of the study were to determine the sensitivity, specificity, and predictive value of screening tools and whether screening reduced site-specific mortality rates. The sample included 37,000 men screened for prostate cancer with DRE and PSA testing who were matched with the same number of unscreened men. Follow-up of these men continued through 2007. Preliminary results reveal that 98.7% of men with an initial PSA value of less than or equal to 1 ng/ml would continue to have PSA levels below 4 ng/ml at the next four annual screenings, thus suggesting that screening for this group could be performed less often. Additionally, 24% of men with an initial PSA value of 2–3 ng/ml were likely to have an elevated level in one year, and 83% were likely to have an elevated level in four years.

Factors That Influence Screening

A number of factors are believed to influence men's participation in prostate cancer screening programs. Traditionally,

lack of access to adequate health care has long been blamed for poor screening efforts among low-income and minority patient populations. Bach et al. (2002) reported that when African American males receive cancer treatment and medical care similar to Caucasian males, disease outcomes are similar. Sanchez, Bowen, Hart, and Spigner (2007) identified several cultural factors that were involved with decision making for prostate cancer screening among African American men. Six focus groups consisting of men 40–70 years old yielded eight themes: knowledge of prostate cancer and clinical services; prostate cancer as a threat to manhood; screening as a threat to manhood; self-awareness of health and well-being; value of screening; convenience of PSA screening; misunderstanding of screening controversy; and distrust of the medical community.

Lack of health insurance also contributes to poor screening participation. Although Medicare coverage is available for men older than age 50 to be screened, it is not required; thus, many states do not have laws mandating that insurers provide coverage for PSA testing (ACS, 2007).

Positive factors shown to influence screening practices include having a friend or family member recently diagnosed with the disease (McKee, 1994). Additionally, African American males were more likely to participate in a prostate cancer screening program if an ethnic role model shared his personal perspective on the importance of screening and when individualized educational interventions were used (Weinrich et al., 1998). When screenings took place in a community setting with participation and organization by active community leaders, participants were more likely to return on a yearly basis (Starr, Waldman, Tester, Kinsey, & Smith, 2002). Results from a pilot study of 10 couples' preferences about prostate cancer screening suggested that women may influence men's attitudes on prostate screening. The majority of husbands in this study were found to prefer no screening, whereas almost all wives preferred screening for their husbands (Volk et al., 2004). More recently, a cross-sectional study of 280 unaffected men with a family history of prostate cancer along with 174 of their partners were surveyed to assess the role of the partners and other factors in influencing prostate cancer screening (Meiser et al., 2007). Factors that influenced willingness to participate in DRE were older age and perception of prostate cancer risk. Additionally, men with sons were more likely to participate in DRE. One significant factor that influenced willingness to undergo PSA screening was the partner's overall involvement in the participant's health maintenance (Meiser et al.).

Screening also has a psychological aspect to consider. Pain, suffering, and psychological distress are components of newly diagnosed prostate cancer (Menhert, Lehmann, Schulte, & Koch, 2007). Men may experience high levels of anxiety while awaiting results from a screening program. This anxiety may enter into their activities of daily living and affect their work and personal relationships (Beebe-Dimmer et al., 2004). The impact of false-positive screening is significant as well, as anxiety associated with cancer may increase and interfere with one's ability to sleep, cause nausea and vomiting, and affect overall quality of life (Linn, Ball, & Maradiegue, 2007).

Screening Tools

Prostate-Specific Antigen Testing

The initial practice and subsequent controversy related to prostate cancer screening has focused on PSA level and what that value means in terms of presence of disease and its diagnostic stage. PSA is a glycoprotein that occurs from prostate cells and is found in higher concentrations in the gland itself than in the peripheral blood. When the integrity of the gland is compromised, elevated levels of PSA can be detected in the bloodstream. Invasive procedures such as biopsy, urethral irritation, and rectal examination can cause a "false" elevation of PSA values. Benign prostatic hypertrophy (BPH) also can cause an abnormally elevated PSA level. Additionally, ejaculation within 48 hours prior to sampling can cause a rise in PSA level (NCCN, 2007). Also, slight elevations in PSA levels have been found to occur after the first few hours of a DRE (Loeb & Catalona, 2007). Thus, PSA elevation alone does not necessarily indicate prostate cancer. If not the result of sexual stimulation or an invasive procedure, PSA elevation may indicate prostate disease, including BPH or infectious prostatitis. PSA testing alone is not specific enough to indicate the presence of prostate cancer. Therefore, DRE should be done in conjunction with PSA testing, and in some cases, transrectal ultrasound (TRUS) may be helpful in evaluating the prostate gland. Also, the patient's symptoms and associated risk factors play an important part in screening for prostate cancer. In 1997, the U.S. Food and Drug Administration approved PSA testing along with DRE for use in the detection of prostate cancer in men 50 years of age and older. Since that time, a number of PSA-based tests have been developed and studied for their clinical significance. Additional information regarding PSA-based testing is available in Chapter 2.

Further consideration regarding PSA testing must be given to age- and race-related PSA reference ranges. Differences in PSA levels and disease stage upon diagnosis have been well studied in African American men, with a higher prevalence of more aggressive disease and higher PSA levels at diagnosis occurring in African Americans than in Caucasians (Moul et al., 1995; Presti, Hovey, Bhargava, Carroll, & Shinohara, 1997). In a retrospective review of 404 Hispanic men and 341 Caucasian men with elevated PSA levels and abnormal DRE, a higher proportion of Hispanic men with serum PSA levels of 2.5–10 ng/ml had prostate cancer, and significantly higher prebiopsy PSA levels were seen in the Hispanic men with positive biopsies than negative biopsies (Lam, Cheung, Benson, & Goluboff, 2003). However, earlier studies showed either no difference between the two groups or lower PSA levels in Hispanic men (Abdalla, Ray, Ray, Vaida, & Vijayakumar, 1998; Canto & Chu, 2000), thus making the broad use of standard PSA ranges across all ethnicities challenging.

Standard PSA reference ranges seem to be less sensitive when compared to age-specific reference ranges, especially for men younger than 60, and seem to be a more specific marker for men older than 60 (Coley, Barry, & Mulley, 1997). Increasing the sensitivity of PSA testing in younger men may allow for the detection of organ-confined disease, and increasing the specificity of the test in older men may avoid unnecessary biopsies (Oesterling, 1995). However, age-specific reference ranges developed for Caucasian men showed poor sensitivity when applied to African American men. In one study, higher PSA values were found among African American men, and the values were more widely distributed among older men (Morgan et al., 1996). Cooney et al. (2001) suggested that minor differences in PSA reference ranges between African American and Caucasian men may not be of sufficient magnitude to recommend the use of race-specific PSA reference ranges for screening.

A number of researchers have suggested adherence to age- and race-specific PSA reference ranges, whereas others advocate adherence to standard testing with a PSA level of 4 ng/ml as the end point for recommending biopsy. In 2000, the American Urological Association PSA Best Practice Task

Force identified age-adjusted PSA, free-to-total PSA, and PSA density as methods to improve PSA specificity (see Chapter 2 for tables showing age- and race-specific PSA levels). Continued use of age- and race-specific PSA reference ranges is hoped to decrease the number of false-positive test results (Olson et al., 1994).

Another consideration in regard to PSA screening is one's PSA velocity (PSAV), which essentially is the absolute increase in the PSA level from an earlier time to a later time (Etzioni, Ankerst, Weiss, Inoue, & Thompson, 2007). PSAV in terms of prognosis is addressed later in this chapter. Carter et al. (2006) theorized that the rate at which PSA levels change may be an important indicator for the presence of life-threatening disease. This study evaluated the relative risks of prostate cancer death and prostate cancer survival stratified by PSAV in three groups of men (N = 980). PSAV measured 10–15 years before diagnosis (when most men had PSA levels below 4 ng/ml) was associated with cancer-specific survival 25 years later; survival was 92% (95% confidence interval [CI] = 84%–96%) among men with PSAV of 0.35 ng/ml per year or less and 54% (95% CI = 15%–82%) among men with PSAV greater than 0.35 ng/ml per year (p < .001). Additionally, men with PSAV greater than 0.35 ng/ml per year had a higher relative risk of prostate cancer death than men with PSAV of 0.35 ng/ml per year or less (relative risk [RR] = 4.7; 95% CI = 1.3–16.5; p = .02). The rates per 100,000 person-years were 1,240 for men with PSAV greater than 0.35 ng/ml per year and 140 for men with PSAV less than or equal to 0.35 ng/ml per year.

Digital Rectal Exam

In addition to PSA-based testing, DRE, although limited as an assessment tool, is an integral part of any prostate cancer screening protocol. However, when used alone, DRE has been shown to have missed approximately 40% of cancers detected during initial screenings (Catalona et al., 1994). In terms of screening, some have argued that DRE should be used only in conjunction with PSA testing. The strength in DRE screening is that it allows clinicians to make PSA screening more selective, thus reducing overdiagnosis. Some physicians believe that DRE may increase the number of diagnoses by adding positive DRE tests to positive PSA tests (Centers for Disease Control and Prevention, 2006). Clinicians skilled in detecting gland abnormalities should perform the DRE. Despite clinician skill and experience, rectal palpation of the anterior and midline portion of the gland is not possible; thus, the potential exists for tumors in these regions to go undetected. DRE assesses for irregular lesions, texture, and symmetry of the gland.

Transrectal Ultrasound

Although it is conceivable that TRUS can be used in conjunction with PSA testing and DRE for screening purposes, it usually is not part of a routine screening program. The primary use of TRUS is to guide needle biopsy and needle placement during prostate brachytherapy. TRUS can confirm abnormal shape and excessive size of the prostate gland. However, nodular irregularities on the prostate gland cannot always be confirmed by TRUS. Clinician experience and expertise significantly influence TRUS interpretation (Waldman, 2006).

Risk Factors

A PSA level is only one determinant of prostate cancer risk. A number of other factors, such as age, race/ethnicity, and family history, have been implicated in influencing prostate cancer risk. It is not totally clear how the interaction of all these variables actually influences overall risk of disease. One study, however, suggested that higher PSA level, positive family history, and abnormal DRE were predictive of developing prostate cancer. Additionally, higher PSA level, abnormal DRE, older age at biopsy, and African American race were predictive of developing high-grade disease (Thompson et al., 2006).

Age

Prostate cancer is by far a disease of older males. Although anecdotal reports exist, the occurrence of prostate cancer before the age of 40 is rare. When it does occur in this age group, it generally behaves in an aggressive manner. Incidence rates increase exponentially after the age of 40 and begin to decline when men reach their 80s. The incidence after age 50 increases on a yearly basis to reach approximately 1,000 cases per 100,000 males aged 65–69. Prostate cancer has been theorized to be a normal part of the aging process, and living to an older age puts men at higher risk of developing the disease (O'Rourke, 2005; Ries et al., 2007).

Race

Incidence rates for prostate cancer in the United States range from 51.2 per 100,000 among Native Americans/Alaska Natives to 271.3 per 100,000 among African American males. Five-year relative survival rates also are lower for African American males than for Caucasians diagnosed with the disease (NCI, 2004). Theories as to the reason for these disparities range from inequalities in access to health care, to whether quality health care is received, to the existence of comorbidities. As previously discussed, some research has suggested that when African Americans receive cancer treatment and medical care similar to Caucasian males, disease outcomes are similar (Bach et al., 2002).

Another theory contends that higher testosterone levels among African American males may be a contributing factor. Serum testosterone levels are, on average, 15% higher among African American males than in Caucasian males. One study examined the relationship between male hormone levels and rates of prostate cancer. The researchers found that dihydrotestosterone (DHT)-testosterone ratios highly corresponded to prostate cancer rates among African Americans, had intermediate correspondence in Caucasians, and had lowest correspondence in Asian Americans (Wu et al., 1995). However, Sofikerim, Eskicorapci, Oruc, and Ozen (2007) suggested that patients diagnosed with prostate cancer have low levels of serum testosterone and high levels of serum follicle-stimulating hormone compared with the patients with BPH. Little evidence was found for the theory that high levels of testosterone increase prostate cancer risk, suggesting that further studies are needed to clarify the relationship between hormones, race, and prostate cancer etiology.

Outside the United States, prostate cancer is common in Africa, and lower rates exist among Asian countries. However, as inhabitants of traditional Eastern countries adopt a more Western lifestyle, prostate cancer rates seem to be rising (Hsing, Tsao, & Devesa, 2000). Interestingly, migration studies also indicate a rise in prostate cancer risk among Asians upon immigration to North America (Shimizu et al., 1991; Whittemore et al., 1995). More recently, the incidence of prostate cancer has risen in a number of Asian countries. Although still much lower than in many Western nations, prostate cancer rates have increased by as much as 102% in Japan and 118% among Chinese men in Singapore. Although overall the low prostate cancer rates among Asians may be attributed to genetic factors, gradual Westernization may be causing many Asian countries to lose their cultural protective factors and acquire factors of higher risk (Sim & Cheng, 2005).

Family History

Family history is a strong risk factor for prostate cancer. Family and twin studies have provided significant evidence to support a hereditary link to prostate cancer, and these studies also have opened the door to extensive research into whether a genetic link or an inherited genetic susceptibility exists for the disease. Two separate meta-analyses have been performed, both of which supported the familial history link (Johns & Houlston, 2003; Zeegers, Jellema, & Ostrer, 2003). The studies reported that the odds ratio for contracting the disease was greater if a brother was affected than the ratio for those with an affected father. Men with only an affected second-degree relative had a lower risk, and recurrence risk was higher when the patient and affected family member were older than 65 years of age (Johns & Houlston; Zeegers et al.). Family history is a potentially greater risk factor for patients younger than 55 than for patients older than 70 (Walsh & Partin, 1997). African American males whose father or brother was diagnosed with prostate cancer at an early age appear to have an even greater risk of developing the disease. Other studies examining a mixed population also support a familial risk

component among various ethnic populations (Cunningham et al., 2003; Whittemore et al., 1995; Zeegers et al.).

Genetics

Although the pathophysiology of prostate cancer is fairly well understood, the underlying molecular defect that triggers malignancy within the prostate gland remains inconclusive. A number of genetic anomalies may be to blame for the multiple ways in which the disease behaves. Genetic changes occur over time related to oncogene expression, deletion of chromosome arms, suppression of apoptosis, activation of oncogenes, and inactivation of tumor suppressor genes. See Table 3-2 for a selected list of somatic gene alterations implicated in prostate carcinogenesis (Clayton, 2006; Linehan, Zbar, Leach, Cordon-Cardo, & Isaacs, 2001).

Table 3-2. Selected Somatic Gene Alterations Associated With Prostate Cancer

Gene	Chromosome Location	Proposed Function
AR	Xq11-12	Binding of androgens and translocation to nucleus for DNA binding; transactivation of gene with androgen responsive elements
CYP17	10q24.3	Testicular synthesis of androgens
SRD5A2	2q23	Catalyzes the irreversible conversion of testosterone to DHT
PTEN	10q23	Inhibits p13/Akt cell-surviving signals
NKX3.1	8p21	Regulates cell growth
GSTP1	11q13	Carcinogen detoxifications
CDKN1B	12p13	Cell cycle control

Note. From "Epidemiology, Risk Factors, and Prevention Strategies," by E.C. Clayton in J. Held-Warmkessel (Ed.), *Contemporary Issues in Prostate Cancer: A Nursing Perspective* (2nd ed., p. 5), 2006, Sudbury, MA: Jones and Bartlett. Copyright 2006 by Jones and Bartlett. Reprinted with permission.

Significant research has been conducted on the androgen DHT and its effect on the intracellular androgen receptor (AR) located on the X chromosome. Upon binding at this site, the DHT-AR complex activates the transcription cascade from within the cell's nucleus (Cheng, Lee, & Grayback, 1993). AR protein activity is related to the length of the CAG repeat. Shorter CAG repeats have been associated with increased AR transcription activity (Beilin, Ball, Favaloro, & Zajac, 2000; Irvine et al., 2000). Shorter CAG repeats in the AR gene usually are found in African American males, thus suggesting a possible cause for a higher incidence of disease among this population (Edwards, Hammond, Jin, Caskey, & Chakraborty, 1992; Irvine, Yu, Ross, & Coetzee, 1995). CAG length also has been implicated in tumor progression. Gene mutations, such as those previously described, have been found among patients with advanced disease (Marcelli et al., 2000).

Hereditary prostate cancer (HPC) typically is characterized by the presence of an autosomal dominant pattern of inheritance and early onset of disease. HPC accounts for approximately 8%–9% of diagnosed cases by age 85 and 43% of cases in men younger than 55 (Verhage et al., 2001; Walsh & Partin, 1997). Several studies, including two meta-analyses, concluded that the risk of developing prostate cancer may be greater if a family member with the disease were a first-degree relative; having a brother with prostate cancer implied greater risk. Second-degree relatives, such as grandfathers or uncles, implied risk but not to the same extent as first-degree relatives (Carter et al., 1993; Johns & Houlston, 2003; Zeegers et al., 2003).

Multiple variants in three regions of chromosome 8q24 consistently have been found to be associated with prostate cancer in population-based association studies. Sun et al. (2008) confirmed that prostate cancer susceptibility exists at 8q24, particularly at region 2, and also provided evidence that this plays an important role in familial prostate cancer. Other studies have examined an inherited genetic susceptibility to prostate cancer by mapping one's genetic markers. HPC1 is found on chromosome 1q, and HPC2 is found on chromosome 17p. HPC20 is found on chromosome 20q, whereas chromosome 8p also has been identified as a gene susceptible to prostate cancer. In fact, multiple susceptibility genes have been identified and continue to be studied for their propensity to cause prostate cancer (DeMarzo, Nelson, Isaacs, & Epstein, 2003; Gronberg et al., 1997; Nelson, DeMarzo, & Isaacs, 2003; Schaid, 2004). Despite these and other studies, only twin and segregation studies have provided evidence for an inherited component to the etiology of prostate cancer. More than a dozen family-based genetic linkage analyses have not been able to consistently identify a genetic susceptibility for prostate cancer (Langeberg, Isaacs, & Stanford, 2007).

Diet

The role of dietary fat and fatty acid intake has been extensively studied over the past two decades, resulting in conflicting reports on the effect that fat intake has on prostate cancer (Attar-Bashi, Frauman, & Sinclair, 2004; Fleshner, Bagnell, Klotz, & Venkateswaran, 2004; Giovannucci et al., 1993; Ramon et al., 2000; Schuurman, van den Brandt, Dorant, Brants, & Goldbohm, 1999). Theories by which dietary fat may increase prostate cancer risk include exposure to fatty acids, increased androgen levels, and oxidative stress. Exposure to fatty acids is suspected to inhibit synthesis of prosta-

glandins, which could negatively affect one's immune system. Countries with the highest per capita fat consumption, such as the United States and those in Western Europe, also have the highest death rates from prostate cancer (Brosman & Moyad, 2008). Fleshner et al. (2004) reviewed the results of several studies that examined the relationship between dietary fat and prostate cancer. They discovered that of the 23 case-control studies describing a positive association, 6 were statistically significant and 7 trended toward significance.

Dietary intake of calcium has been suggestive of an increased risk of prostate cancer. Analysis of data from a prospective cohort study of 51,529 men, known as the Health Professionals Follow-Up Study, showed high intake of calcium (> 2,000 mg versus < 500 mg) was associated with a 4.6-fold increased risk of metastatic prostate cancer (Giovannucci et al., 1998). Similar data from a case-controlled study indicated that calcium intake (> 1,183 mg/day) confers a higher risk of prostate cancer compared with those consuming lower levels of calcium (< 825 mg/day) (Chan et al., 1998). Data from the Cancer Prevention Study II Nutrition Cohort also showed that higher calcium intake was associated with a small but significant increase in prostate cancer risk (Rodriguez et al., 2003). Giovannucci, Liu, Stampfer, and Willet (2006) suggested that calcium intake exceeding 1,500 mg/day may be associated with a decrease in differentiation in prostate cancer and ultimately with a higher risk of advanced and fatal prostate cancer but not with well-differentiated, organ-confined cancers.

Other agents such as vitamins A, D, and E, selenium, phytoestrogens, and pomegranate also have been studied for their relationship to prostate cancer risk. Vitamin A, a fat soluble vitamin that promotes normal cellular growth, has shown little effect (Omenn et al., 1996). Conversely, stronger evidence exists to support a relationship between prostate cancer and the antioxidant vitamin E and selenium (Heinonen et al., 1998; Klein et al., 2001; Virtamo et al., 2003), which is found in prostate enzymes. Calcitriol, a form of vitamin D, has been shown to arrest the G0/G1 phase of meiosis, inhibit angiogenesis, and induce apoptosis (Rackley, Clark, & Hall, 2006). Soy phytoestrogens seem to demonstrate protective effects against prostate cancer (Zhou et al., 1999), and epidemiologic data have suggested that intake of soy may reduce the risk of the disease (Cross et al., 2004; Lee et al., 2003). Handayani et al. (2006) examined Asians with diets high in soy isoflavones to determine if any chemoprotective properties were present. Soy isoflavone concentrate was found to inhibit the growth of PC3 human prostate cancer cells through modulation of cell cycle progression and the expression of genes involved in cell cycle regulation, metastasis, and angiogenesis.

Pantuck et al. (2006) sought to determine the effects of pomegranate juice consumption in men with a rising PSA level following primary surgery or radiation therapy. Forty-six patients were given eight ounces of juice daily until disease progression. Mean PSA doubling time significantly lengthened with pomegranate treatment from a mean of 15 months at baseline to 54 months after treatment ($p < .001$). This study was later updated to reflect continued lengthening of PSA doubling time to 58.4 months, suggesting that pomegranate juice may be beneficial to this subset of patients. A multicenter, randomized, phase III study is ongoing to further evaluate the benefits of pomegranate in a placebo-controlled manner (Pantuck et al., 2008).

Lycopene, a carotenoid found in tomato-based products, also has been reported to have conflicting effects on prostate cancer risk. A number of prospective dietary studies have found that a higher intake of tomato products was associated with a decreased risk (Ansari & Gupta, 2004; Giovannucci, Ascherio, & Rimm, 1995; Kucuk et al., 2001; Mills, Beeson, Phillips, & Fraser, 1989). Alternatively, studies exist that do not support such an association (Hayes et al., 1999; Kolonel et al., 2000; Rackley et al., 2006).

Further research into the role that dietary intake has on prostate cancer risk is needed to validate the numerous hypotheses and suspicions that exist among researchers and the general population.

Alcohol and Smoking

Although alcohol intake has been associated with increased rates of some malignancies, conclusive evidence of a strong correlation with prostate cancer does not exist. Some studies have focused on the amount of alcohol consumed (Putnam et al., 2000; Sesso, Paffenbarger, & Lee, 2001; Albertsen & Gronbaek, 2002; Nilsen, Johnsen, & Vatten, 2000), whereas others have examined the type of alcohol ingested (Platz, Leitzmann, Rimm, Willett, & Giovannucci, 2004; Schuurman, Goldbohm, & van den Brandt, 1999; Sutcliffe et al., 2007; Velicer, Kristal, & White, 2006; Villeneuve, Johnson, Krieger, & Mao, 1999). Overall, alcohol intake does not appear to be a significant risk factor for prostate cancer. On the other hand, some evidence exists to suggest that cigarette smoking may increase one's risk of developing and dying from the disease (Coughlin, Neaton, & Sengupta, 1996; Giovannucci et al., 1999; Gong, Agalliu, Lin, Stanford, & Kristal, 2008; Plaskon, Penson, Vaughan, & Stanford, 2003; Rodriguez, Tatham, Thun, Calle, & Heath, 1997).

Miscellaneous

A number of other factors have been examined for a possible link to prostate cancer, which include hormonal exposure, body mass index, physical activity, occupational/chemical exposure, and issues surrounding male sexuality (e.g., frequency of sexual activity, vasectomy, human papillomavirus exposure) (Clayton, 2006; Held-Warmkessel, 2005). However, little supportive evidence exists that would suggest a strong relationship between these factors and prostate cancer.

Prevention

Relative to its incidence, the mortality rate from prostate cancer is low. However, interest in prostate cancer prevention remains high among healthcare practitioners and the public at large. Prevention strategies generally are considered to be primary, secondary, or tertiary. The goal of primary prevention strategies is to prevent people with no evidence of clinical disease, inclusive of those with premalignant lesions, from developing invasive, life-threatening cancer (Gann & Giovannucci, 2004). Presently, in terms of prostate cancer, this has yet to occur. Over the past few decades, significant research has identified genetic and environmental risk factors for prostate cancer, some of which have been previously described in this chapter. However, because of conflicting data or because of an outright lack of data, a clinically useful means to stratify men according to their level of risk for the disease does not exist. Secondary prevention strategies include activities that detect disease early and limit disease effects after diagnosis. In terms of prostate cancer, such strategies would include screening with PSA testing and DRE. Although DRE as a means of secondary prevention may be in question, as only portions of the gland itself are palpable and, as previously described, such an examination is subject to clinician expertise. Tertiary prevention strategies include engaging in activities that prevent further disability and restoring a higher level of functioning in someone with the disease. In terms of prostate cancer, this would include pain control in advanced disease and modalities used in the treatment of the disease, which are discussed in Chapter 4.

Primary prevention strategies are largely targeted at the cellular changes and biochemical processes that occur in carcinogenesis. Prostate carcinogenesis is a multistep process that is initiated with the malignant potential of any one cell. At some point, the malignant potential of a cell becomes real when an accumulation of genetic changes results in a pattern of cellular atypia, deregulation of cell growth, and eventual carcinoma. Because the carcinogenic process is believed to take decades, opportunity exists for early primary preventive interventions when mutations are few (Clayton, 2006; Crawford, 2007). Primary prevention studies to date have included pharmaceutical approaches and dietary/nutritional approaches.

Pharmaceutical Approaches

In a massive accumulation of subjects, the Prostate Cancer Prevention Trial randomly assigned 18,882 asymptomatic men with normal DRE and PSA levels less than 3 ng/ml to placebo or the antiandrogen drug finasteride (Thompson et al., 2003). Throughout the seven years of the study, the men underwent annual DREs and PSA measurements. Because it was known that finasteride lowered PSA levels, all cancer-free men were subjected to biopsy by the end of the study.

Following 5.75 years of follow-up, the study was terminated, and it was found that 81.3% of patients had completed the full seven years of therapy. Of the 9,060 men included in the final analysis, prostate cancer was detected in 18.4% of patients in the finasteride group and in 24.4% of patients in the placebo group, equaling a risk reduction of 24.8%. Of interest was that a greater proportion of patients in the finasteride group were diagnosed with Gleason score (GS) 7–10 tumors. Study results were encouraging in that finasteride reduced the prevalence of prostate cancer, but the higher grade of cancers detected on biopsy brings into question the benefit from finasteride (Gann & Giovannucci, 2004).

Another antiandrogen, dutasteride, currently is being investigated for its preventive potential. The REDUCE (Reduction by Dutasteride of Prostate Cancer Events) trial has enrolled 800 men at least 50 years of age with negative biopsies and PSA level of 2.5–10 ng/ml. Each patient is to receive dutasteride daily and eventually undergo biopsy at two and four years (Thorpe et al., 2007).

Some laboratory data exist to suggest that antiestrogens may be effective at reducing the risk of prostate cancer. A randomized, double-blind trial examined 514 men with high-grade prostate intraepithelial neoplasia and no evidence of prostate cancer on screening biopsy. The men were randomized to receive 20, 40, or 60 mg toremifene or placebos daily for 12 months. The study found that the cumulative risk of prostate cancer was decreased in patients on 20 mg of the study drug versus placebo (24.4% and 31.2%, respectively). The annualized rate of prevention was 6.8 cancers per 100 men treated. In patients with no biopsy evidence of cancer at baseline and 6 months, the 12-month incidence of prostate cancer was decreased by 48.2% with 20 mg toremifene versus placebo (9.1% versus 17.4%, respectively). The 20 mg dose of toremifene was effective, but cumulative and 12-month incidences of prostate cancer were lower for each toremifene dose versus placebo. Upon biopsy review, GSs were similar across each treatment group. Researchers concluded the toremifene decreased the incidence of prostate cancer by one year and had a tolerable side effect profile versus placebo in this high-risk population (Price et al., 2006).

Another class of drugs that was recently examined for its preventive effective on prostate cancer was the cyclooxygenase-2 inhibitors. However, because of concerns regarding the increase in cardiovascular events observed among patients on these drugs, the trials were closed (Clayton, 2006).

Dietary/Nutritional Approaches

Most of the research examining nutritional elements that delay disease development or disease progression has been conducted on lycopene, vitamin E, selenium, and vitamin D. However, numerous studies, including anecdotal reports, have looked at dozens of nutritional agents to prevent prostate cancer. This review will consist of the more recent and promising of these agents.

A number a studies have examined the carotenoid lycopene and tomato-based products. Mills et al. (1989) conducted a multivariate analysis and found that high consumption of peas, lentils, beans, and tomato-based products showed a statistically significant reduction in prostate cancer risk.

In the Health Professionals Follow-Up Study (Giovannucci et al., 1995), researchers reported that high intake of lycopene resulted in a trend toward reduced prostate cancer risk (RR = 0.79; 95% CI = 0.64–0.99; p = .04). Specifically, tomato sauce had the strongest inverse relationship in this study (RR = 0.66; 95% CI = 0.49–0.90; p = .001). In a follow-up study (Giovannucci, Rimm, Liu, Stampfer, & Willett, 2002), results again showed an association of lycopene with reduced prostate cancer risk (RR = 0.84; 95% CI = 0.73–0.96; p = .003).

In a more recent study, Kumar et al. (2008) examined the effect of lycopene on men already diagnosed with clinically localized prostate cancer. In this phase II randomized study, 45 men took 15, 30, or 45 mg of oral lycopene or no supplement for four to six weeks. The researchers found that serum-free testosterone decreased from baseline and total estradiol increased significantly in the 30 mg group. They also observed a statistically significant increase in serum total estradiol and sex hormone and sex hormone–binding globulin in the men treated with 45 mg of lycopene with no significant change in serum-free testosterone. No statistically significant changes occurred in serum PSA level with lycopene supplementation. The researchers concluded that lycopene potentially may reduce prostate cancer risk via the steroid hormone pathway.

Although vitamin E is known to have antioxidant effects, results from clinical trials looking at its preventive properties for prostate cancer may be limited to specific patient populations. The Alpha-Tocopherol, Beta-Carotene (ATBC) Cancer Prevention Study evaluated whether supplementation with alpha-tocopherol, the most active form of vitamin E, or beta-carotene could reduce prostate cancer risk (Heinonen et al., 1998). The ATBC study consisted of more than 29,000 male smokers, as it was originally designed to examine the role of supplementation on lung cancer development and only secondarily on other cancers. Participants were randomized to receive placebo, alpha-tocopherol, beta-carotene, or the combination. Following a median of 6.1 years of follow-up, the alpha-tocopherol group demonstrated a 34% reduction in incidence of prostate cancer versus the placebo group, with a 40% reduction in the incidence of clinically meaningful tumors (stage II–IV) and in prostate cancer–specific mortality. Of note, however, was that a 32% decrease in the incidence of prostate cancer among participants receiving alpha-tocopherol versus placebo was observed after the first year, and no differences were noted in the incidence of latent disease (stage 0–I), suggesting that the role of vitamin E might be best seen in the progression of disease from earlier stages to later stages.

Furthermore, because the study consisted of only smokers, it is questionable whether the results can be generalized to a larger, nonsmoking population. The act of smoking tobacco alone may have had an effect on the study outcomes as well.

More recently, data from the Physicians Health Study II regarding vitamins A and C was presented at the 7th Annual International Conference on Frontiers in Cancer Prevention Research. The study was a large scale, long-term, randomized trial that included more than 14,500 physicians who were at least 50 years of age at enrollment. Over a 10-year period, participants were randomized to either 400 IU of vitamin E four times daily or its placebo or 500 mg of vitamin C or its placebo. Analyses indicate that neither vitamin E nor vitamin C supplementation produced significant evidence to suggest a reduction in the incidence of prostate cancer, or any other kind of cancer, for that matter. Another component of the study examining the effects of multivitamin supplementation is ongoing (American Association for Cancer Research, 2008).

It is hoped that additional information gained from the Selenium and Vitamin E Cancer Prevention Trial (SELECT) will provide more evidence as to whether the effects of vitamin E are seen only in specific patient populations. This prospective trial has randomized 32,400 men to placebo, selenium alone (200 mcg/day), alpha-tocopherol alone (400 mg/day), or a combination of both for a minimum of 7 years and a maximum of 12 (Klein et al., 2003). Some early studies with selenium alone and its synergistic properties with vitamin E have shown promising results in preventing prostate cancer and reducing cancer in prostate cancer cell lines (Clark et al., 1998; Venkateswaran, Fleshner, & Klotz, 2004; Yoshizawa et al., 1998). Results of the SELECT trial are not expected until 2012.

Research examining pharmacologic and nutritional preventive strategies for prostate cancer is relatively new, and additional follow-up studies are needed to identify conclusive links. Development of studies to confer positive and negative effects on prostate cancer development is needed, as is investigation into new and unexamined agents. As information from ongoing trials becomes available, healthcare professionals can act to influence change in patients' diets and lifestyles to decrease their risk of developing prostate cancer.

New trials that are under way through NCI that examine the preventive effects of nutrition on prostate cancer include trial numbers NCT00322114 (lycopene), NCT00253643 (fish oil supplements in men with prostatic intraepithelial neoplasia [PIN]), and NCT00118066 (phase II trial of calcitriol in men with high-grade PIN) (NCI, 2008).

Prognosis

The purpose of accurate prognosis is to enhance the healthcare practitioner's ability to counsel patients regarding survival and treatment options along with their associated risks and benefits. Accurate prognosis also allows patients to make informed decisions regarding treatment options and desired quality of life. Disease progression of prostate cancer is determined by histologic grade of tumor, clinical disease stage, and PSA level. Historically, three particular nomograms have been used and are reported in the literature. Each nomogram is used independent of the others, and each considers grade of tumor, clinical stage of disease, and PSA level. Nomograms commonly are used to determine the probability of a particular clinical end point (Carter, DeMarzo, & Lilja, 2004).

Traditional Models

The Partin tables combine the American Joint Committee on Cancer (AJCC) tumor stage, GS, and serum PSA level to preoperatively predict the final pathologic stage of the tumor. Independent validation of the Partin tables demonstrated that they correctly predict pathologic stage of a tumor in 70%–80% of cases (Augustin et al., 2004). Of specific concern in tumor staging is whether the disease is confined to the prostate or if it has extended to the seminal vesicles or surrounding lymph nodes (Partin et al., 1993). Unfortunately, the Partin tables are unable to account for individual pathologic features such as seminal vesicle invasion irrespective of lymph node status because the pathologic stage that includes seminal vesicle invasion assumes negative lymph node status (Kattan, 2007). Three versions of the Partin tables have been published, in 1993, 1997, and 2001. The most recent version was later updated by Makarov et al. (2007) using data from patients treated between 2000 and 2005 to reflect an up-to-date patient population.

The D'Amico model examines preoperative PSA level, GS, and AJCC tumor stage to predict 10-year PSA failure-free survival in patients with localized prostate cancer who undergo radical prostatectomy. This model may help to identify patients who are less likely to remain disease-free and therefore are more suited for additional treatment or possible enrollment in a clinical trial (D'Amico, 2001). D'Amico's research examined 2,127 patients and reported that the estimated 10-year PSA failure-free survival was 83% for those considered to be at low risk, 46% in patients considered to be at intermediate risk, and 29% in men considered to be at high risk. However, prediction of biochemical failure at 10 years is not necessarily reflective of mortality, as many patients live for many years following PSA failure (Carter et al., 2004).

The Kattan nomogram uses data from postoperative prostatectomy patients to evaluate the long-term probability of disease recurrence to help to determine the appropriate use of adjuvant therapies. Kattan, Eastham, Stapleton, Wheeler, and Scardino (1998) examined serum PSA level, degree of capsular invasion, GS, surgical margin status, seminal vesicle invasion, and lymph node status in 996 patients with T1a–T3c disease. The probability of freedom from failure was 73% at five years. The predicted probability from the nomogram compared with the actual outcome showed a concordance of 0.88. However, in a subsequent validation study, an overall concordance factor of 0.68 was realized, and it was reported that the Kattan nomogram overestimated recurrence-free survival in patients who were at lower risk (Greene et al., 2004).

Different from a predictive nomogram for clinical outcomes, the CaPSURE™ (Cancer of the Prostate Strategic Urologic Research Endeavor) study developed a model that examined quality-of-life issues, such as continence, potency, and physical and mental health outcomes at one year after prostatectomy. Clinical stage of disease, PSA level, and GS were not used as baseline data. Instead, age, income, and fewer comorbidities were independent predictors of quality of life. Furthermore, patients without comorbidities and with good self-reported health status were found to be more likely to return to baseline physical and mental health (Hu et al., 2004).

Serum-Based Practice

More recently, prognosis models have been moving away from traditional nomograms and toward indicators of improved outcome predictions in patients with localized prostate cancer, such as changes in PSA level, and computer software programs. Of specific interest in terms of improved prognosis are changing PSA values, specifically PSAV and PSA doubling time. Again, PSAV is essentially the absolute increase in the PSA level from an earlier time to a later time. PSA doubling time is the amount of time it takes for PSA values to double in any one particular patient (Etzioni et al., 2007). However, these values alone have not been associated with improved screening outcomes, and current screening guidelines put forth by NCCN propose that PSAV be used in combination with PSA testing. However, both measures have been associated with increased risk of adverse clinical outcomes (metastatic disease and prostate cancer–specific mortality) after initial treatment for prostate cancer (Spurgeon et al., 2007).

Loeb, Roehl, Yu, Han, and Catalona (2007) set out to identify a link between increased PSAV and a diagnosis of prostate cancer among men with high-grade PIN. PSAV values of 190 men from screening programs were compared to the PSAV values of men who later developed prostate cancer and those who did not. Median PSAV was significantly greater in the men with high-grade PIN who were subsequently diagnosed with prostate cancer (p = .03). A PSA threshold of 0.75 ng/ml/year predicted which men with high-grade PIN would ultimately be diagnosed with cancer of the prostate (p = .007). On multivariate analysis, including PSAV, age, and initial PSA level, PSAV was the only significant predictor of eventual prostate cancer detection.

In another study, PSAV was examined among 1,095 men with stage T1c or T2 prostate cancer for five years following radical prostatectomy. Compared with patients who had an annual PSAV value of less than 2 ng/ml, an annual PSAV value of greater than 2 ng/ml in the year before resection was significantly associated with lymph node metastases,

advanced pathologic stage, and high-grade disease. In addition, patients with higher rates of PSAV were significantly more likely to develop biochemical disease recurrence, to experience death from prostate cancer, and to experience death from any cause (D'Amico, Chen, Roehl, & Catalona, 2004).

Pinsky et al. (2007) also examined the relationship between PSAV and prostate cancer GS and stage of disease. Data were analyzed from 1,441 men enrolled in the Prostate, Lung, Colorectal, and Ovarian Cancer Screening Trial who received two or more PSA screening tests and were subsequently diagnosed with prostate cancer within one year from the last screen. In this study, PSAV values were estimated by using all screening PSA values within six years before the diagnosis. The results showed that PSA and PSAV values were related to biopsy GS. Multivariate odds ratios for having a GS of 7–10 were 1.3 (95% CI = 0.9–1.9), 2.2 (95% CI = 1.5–3.3), and 2.3 (95% CI = 1.4–3.9) for men with a PSAV values of 0.5–1 ng/ml/year, 1–2 ng/ml/year, and greater than 2 ng/ml/year, respectively, compared with men who had PSAV values less than 0.5 ng/ml/year. The median PSAV value was 0.60 ng/ml/year for men with GSs 2–6, versus 0.84 ng/ml/year for men with GSs 7–10 (p < .0001). The study further examined 658 men who went on to prostatectomy and found that PSA and PSAV values were associated with advanced pathologic stage. However, when controls were implemented for clinical stage and biopsy GS, the associations of PSA and PSAV values were no longer statistically significant for men in the prostatectomy cohort.

In terms of PSA doubling time, studies have shown that a doubling time of less than 10 months has been associated with an increased risk of local recurrence of disease, metastatic progression, and death (Cannon, Walsh, Partin, & Pound, 2003; Pound et al., 1999). In these studies, PSA doubling time was found to be an independent predictor of time to development of metastatic disease when added to other variables such as GS and time to biochemical progression.

A review of 8,669 patients with localized or locally advanced, nonmetastatic disease reported that a PSA doubling time of less than three months was shown to predict death from prostate cancer following radical prostatectomy or radiation therapy (D'Amico, 2007).

The utility of PSAV and PSA doubling time, in terms of prognosis, continues to be examined among many different cohorts who have prostate cancer. Such research is important in identifying the most practical use of these PSA measurements and how they compare to other methods used for prognosis and disease progression, including traditional nomograms, regression analysis, and computer software programs.

Software-Based Models

Artificial neural networks (ANNs) are software programs that build predictive models by weighing multiple factors

CHAPTER 3. PROSTATE CANCER SCREENING, RISK, PREVENTION, AND PROGNOSIS

and comparing them with standardized cases and known outcomes (Crawford, 2003). Such programs are capable of generating data-driven models without making assumptions on statistical distributions (Abbod, Catto, Linkens, & Hamdy, 2007). In 2001, an ANN was developed to predict lymph node spread in patients from two institutions with stage T1a–T3a prostate cancer. The model identified approximately 80% as having a low risk of lymph node spread, with a 2% false-negative rate using clinical T stage, GS, and preoperative PSA level (Batuello et al., 2001). It has been suggested that compared to traditional regression statistics, artificial intelligence methods appear to be more accurate and more explorative for analyzing large data cohorts while allowing for individualized prediction of disease (Abbod et al.). However, Chun et al. (2007) performed a critical appraisal for accuracy of regression-based nomograms, ANNs, regression-tree models, and look-up tables in risk groups for prostate cancer. Although the researchers determined that ANNs are methodologically sound, they suggested that nomograms are more accurate and have better performance characteristics than the other examined alternatives, including ANNs.

ANNs also have been used to predict risk for initial prostate biopsy outcome predictions and recurrence and long-term survival following prostatectomy, as well as in numerous other malignancies. Further refinement of ANNs is needed, as are additional comparative studies to determine whether traditional predictive models can be replaced or if the role of this emerging technology is better suited for specific cohorts and perhaps as an adjunct to previously described prognostic measures.

Individualized Prognostic Approach

The multiple variables that must be considered, as well as the ability of current nomograms and ANNs to generalize and accurately predict outcomes, complicate the current challenge of predicting individual patient risk and prognosis. Risk can be assessed either at the time of diagnosis or after definitive treatment. Even with the most complete of nomograms and advanced programming of artificial intelligence, each method is hampered by limitations that prohibit personalized predictive testing of prostate cancer risk assessment. A relatively new and highly complex method of predicting personalized patient outcomes following treatment for prostate cancer is an approach known as systems pathology. This approach integrates individualized patient-specific information from tissue architecture, clinical data, and the cellular localization and quantification of molecular information. Tissue architecture is obtained for statistical purposes and is performed by way of high-resolution digital imagery at the cellular level. Clinical data include analysis of GS, pathologic stage, and PSA values. The molecular information is gained through multiplexed in situ protein detection using fluorescently tagged antibodies

and analysis via spectral imaging (Alter, 2007; Saidi, Cordon-Cardo, & Costa, 2007).

Additional research on highly individualized assessment models is needed to determine the predictive capability of disease progression and accuracy, as well as improved risk discrimination, versus other more traditional and commonly used methods of prognostic assessment.

Conclusion

Issues surrounding prostate cancer screening, risk factors associated with the disease, prevention strategies, and prognostic indicators continue to evolve. Controversies continue to exist in terms of screening practice both in the United States and worldwide. PSA-based testing is the most recognized form of screening and is the most often used method of tracking response to treatment. However, the most optimal form of PSA-based testing continues to be debated. As the natural history of prostate cancer continues to unfold and clinical trial data are accumulated, oncology practitioners will be in a better position to counsel patients and caregivers as to the best practice in terms of screening and treatment.

References

Abbod, M.F., Catto, J.W., Linkens, D.A., & Hamdy, F.C. (2007). Application of artificial intelligence to the management of urological cancer. *Journal of Urology, 178*(4, Pt. 1), 1150–1156.

Abdalla, I., Ray, P., Ray, V., Vaida, F., & Vijayakumar, S. (1998). Comparison of serum prostate specific antigen levels and PSA density in African-American, white, and Hispanic men without prostate cancer. *Urology, 51*(2), 300–305.

Albertsen, K., & Gronbaek, M. (2002). Does the amount or type of alcohol influence prostate cancer risk? *Prostate, 52*(4), 297–304.

Alter, J.M. (2007). Prostate cancer risk assessment: Personalized, predictive testing is the future. *Oncology Nursing News, 1*(3), 15–16.

American Association for Cancer Research. (2008). *No protective effect on cancer from long-term vitamin E or vitamin C supplementation.* Retrieved November 18, 2008, from http://www.aacr .org/home/public--media/news.aspx?d=1175

American Academy of Family Physicians. (2008, March). *Summary of recommendations for clinical preventive services* [AAFP policy action revision 6.5]. Retrieved July 11, 2008, from http://www .aafp.org/online/en/home/clinical/clinicalrecs.html

American Cancer Society. (2007). *Prostate cancer: Early detection.* Retrieved March 21, 2008, from http://www.cancer.org/docroot/ CRI/content/CRI_2_6x_Prostate_Cancer_Early_Detection .asp?sitearea=

American Cancer Society. (2008, March 5). *American Cancer Society guidelines for the early detection of cancer.* Retrieved March 7, 2008, from http://www.cancer.org/docroot/PED/ content/PED_2_3X_ACS_Cancer_Detection_Guidelines_36 .asp?sitearea=PED

American College of Physicians. (1997). Clinical guideline: Part III: Screening for prostate cancer. *Annals of Internal Medicine, 126*(6), 480–484.

American Medical Association. (2001). *Featured report: Screening and early detection of prostate cancer* [Resolution 511 (I-99)]. Retrieved March 21, 2008, from http://www.ama-assn.org/ama/pub/category/13604.html

Andriole, G.L., Levin, D.L., Crawford, E.D., Gelmann, E.P., Pinsky, P.F., Chia, D., et al. (2005). Prostate cancer screening in the prostate, lung, colorectal and ovarian (PLCO) cancer screening trial: Findings from the initial screening round of a randomized trial. *Journal of the National Cancer Institute, 97*(6), 433–438.

Ansari, M.S., & Gupta, N.P. (2004). Lycopene: A novel drug therapy in hormone refractory metastatic prostate cancer. *Urologic Oncology, 22*(5), 415–420.

Attar-Bashi, N.M., Frauman, A.G., & Sinclair, A.J. (2004). Alpha-linolenic acid and the risk of prostate cancer: What is the evidence? *Journal of Urology, 171*(4), 1402–1407.

Augustin, H., Eggert, T., Wenske, S., Karakiewicz, P.I., Palisaar, J., Daghofer, F., et al. (2004). Comparison of accuracy between the Partin tables of 1997 and 2001 to predict final pathological stage in clinically localized prostate cancer. *Journal of Urology, 171*(1), 177–181.

Bach, P.B., Schrag, D., Brawley, O.W., Galaznik, A., Yakren, S., & Begg, C.B. (2002). Survival of blacks and whites after a cancer diagnosis. *JAMA, 287*(16), 2106–2112.

Batuello, J.T., Gamito, E.J., Crawford, E.D., Han, M., Partin, A.W., McLeod, D.G., et al. (2001). Artificial neural network model for the assessment of lymph node spread in patients with clinically localized prostate cancer. *Urology, 57*(3), 481–485.

Beebe-Dimmer, J.L., Wood, D.P., Gruber, S.B., Chilson, D.M., Zuhlke, K.A., Claeys, G.B., et al. (2004). Risk perception and concern among brothers of men with prostate carcinoma. *Cancer, 100*(7), 1537–1544.

Beilin, J., Ball, E.M., Favaloro, J.M., & Zajac, J.D. (2000). Effect of androgen receptor CAG repeat polymorphism on transcriptional activity: Specificity in prostate and non-prostate cell lines. *Journal of Molecular Endocrinology, 25*(1), 85–96.

Brosman, S.A., & Moyad, M. (2008, February). *Prostate cancer: Nutrition.* Retrieved July 11, 2008, from http://www.emedicine.com/med/topic3100.htm#section~DietaryFatandProstateCancer

Cannon, G.M., Walsh, P.C., Partin, A.W., & Pound, C.L. (2003). Prostate-specific antigen doubling time in the identification of patients at risk for progression after treatment and biochemical recurrence for prostate cancer. *Urology, 62*(Suppl. 2B), 2–8.

Canto, M.T., & Chu, K.C. (2000). Annual cancer incidence rates for Hispanics in the United States: Surveillance, epidemiology and end-results 1992–1996. *Cancer, 88*(11), 2642–2652.

Carter, B.S., Bova, G.S., Beaty, T.H., Steinberg, G.D., Childs, B., Isaacs, W.B., et al. (1993). Hereditary prostate cancer: Epidemiologic and clinical features. *Journal of Urology, 150*(3), 797–802.

Carter, H.B., DeMarzo, A., & Lilja, H. (2004, September). Detection, diagnosis, and prognosis of prostate cancer. In Prostate Cancer Foundation, *Report to the nation on prostate on prostate cancer 2004.* Retrieved February 26, 2008, from http://www.medscape.com/viewprogram/3440

Carter, H.B., Ferrucci, L., Kettermann, A., Landis, P., Wright, E.J., Epstein, J.I., et al. (2006). Detection of life-threatening prostate cancer with prostate-specific antigen velocity during a window of curability. *Journal of the National Cancer Institute, 98*(21), 1521–1527.

Catalona, W.J., Richie, J.P., Ahmann, F.R., Hudson, M.A., Scardino, P.T., Flanigan, R.C., et al. (1994). Comparison of digital rectal examination and serum prostate specific antigen in the early detection of prostate cancer: Results of a multicenter clinical trial of 6630 men. *Journal of Urology, 151*(5), 1283–1290.

Centers for Disease Control and Prevention. (2006, September). *Prostate cancer conference report session 3: Secondary prevention and treatment.* Retrieved March 10, 2008, from http://www.cdc.gov/cancer/prostate/publications/prosfuture/session3.htm

Chan, J.M., Giovannucci, E., Andersson, S.O., Yuen, J., Adami, H.O., & Wolk, A. (1998). Dairy products, calcium, phosphorous, vitamin D, and risk of prostate cancer (Sweden). *Cancer Causes and Control, 9*(6), 559–566.

Cheng, E., Lee, C., & Grayback, J. (1993). Endocrinology of the prostate. In H. Lepor & R.K. Lawson (Eds.), *Prostate diseases* (pp. 57–71). Philadelphia: Saunders.

Chun, F.K., Karakiewicz, P.I., Briganti, A., Walz, J., Kattan, M.W., Huland, H., et al. (2007). A critical appraisal of logistic regression-based nomograms, artificial neural networks, classification and regression-tree models, look-up tables and risk-group stratification models for prostate cancer. *BJU International, 99*(4), 794–800.

Clark, L.C., Dalkin, B., Krongrad, A., Combs, G.F., Turnbull, B.W., Slate, E.H., et al. (1998). Decreased incidence of prostate cancer with selenium supplementation: Results of a double-blind cancer prevention trial. *British Journal of Urology, 81*(5), 730–734.

Clayton, E.C. (2006). Epidemiology, risk factors, and prevention strategies. In J. Held-Warmkessel (Ed.), *Contemporary issues in prostate cancer: A nursing perspective* (2nd ed., pp. 1–43). Sudbury, MA: Jones and Bartlett.

Coley, C.M., Barry, M.J., & Mulley, A.G. (1997). Clinical guideline: Part III: Screening for prostate cancer. *Annals of Internal Medicine, 126*(6), 480–484.

Cooney, K.A., Strawderman, M.S., Wojno, K.J., Doerr, K.M., Taylor, A., Alcser, K.H., et al. (2001). Age-specific distribution of serum prostate-specific antigen in a community-based study of African-American men. *Urology, 57*(1), 91–96.

Coughlin, S.S., Neaton, J.D., & Sengupta, A. (1996). Cigarette smoking as a predictor of death from prostate cancer in 348,874 men screened for the Multiple Risk Factor Intervention Trial. *American Journal of Epidemiology, 143*(10), 1002–1006.

Crawford, E.D. (2003). Use of algorithms as determinants for individual patient decision making: National Comprehensive Cancer Network versus artificial neural networks. *Urology, 62*(6, Suppl. 1), 13–19.

Crawford, E.D. (2007). *Chemoprevention strategies in prostate cancer.* Retrieved January 20, 2008, from http://patients.uptodate.com/topic.asp?file=prost_ca/8237

Cross, H.S., Kallay, E., Lechner, D., Gerdenitsch, W., Adlercreutz, H., & Armbrecht, H.J. (2004). Phytoestrogens and vitamin D metabolism: A new concept for the prevention and therapy of colorectal, prostate, and mammary carcinomas. *Journal of Nutrition, 134*(5), 1207S–1212S.

Cunningham, G., Ashton, C., Annegers, J., Souchek, J., Klima, M., & Miles, B. (2003). Familial aggregation of prostate cancer in African-Americans and White Americans. *Prostate, 56*(4), 256–262.

D'Amico, A. (2007). Global update on defining and treating high-risk localized prostate cancer with leuprorelin: A USA perspective—identifying men at diagnosis who are at high risk of prostate cancer death after surgery or radiation therapy. *BJU International, 99*(Suppl. 1), 13–16, 17–18.

D'Amico, A.V. (2001). Combined-modality staging for localized adenocarcinoma of the prostate. *Oncology (Williston Park), 15*(8), 1049–1059.

D'Amico, A.V., Chen, M.H., Roehl, K.A., & Catalona, W.J. (2004). Preoperative PSA velocity and the risk of death from prostate cancer after radical prostatectomy. *New England Journal of Medicine, 351*(2), 125–135.

DeMarzo, A.M., Nelson, W.G., Isaacs, W.B., & Epstein, J.I. (2003). Pathological and molecular aspects of prostate cancer. *Lancet, 361*(9361), 955–964.

Edwards, A., Hammond, H.A., Jin, L., Caskey, C.T., & Chakraborty, R. (1992). Genetic variation at five trimeric and tetrameric tandem repeat loci in four human population groups. *Genomics, 12*(2), 241–253.

Espey, D.K., Wu, X.C., Swan, J., Wiggins, C., Jim, M.A., Ward, E., et al. (2007). Annual report to the nation on the status of cancer, 1975–2004, featuring cancer in American Indians and Alaska Natives. *Cancer, 110*(10), 2119–2152.

Etzioni, R.D., Ankerst, D.P., Weiss, N.S., Inoue, L.Y.T., & Thompson, I.M. (2007). Is prostate-specific antigen velocity useful in early detection of prostate cancer? A critical appraisal of the evidence. *Journal of the National Cancer Institute, 99*(20), 1510–1515.

Ferrini, R., & Woolf, S.H. (1998). American College of Preventive Medicine practice policy. Screening for prostate cancer in American men. *American Journal of Preventive Medicine, 15*(1), 81–84.

Fleshner, N., Bagnell, P.S., Klotz, L., & Venkateswaran, A. (2004). Dietary fat and prostate cancer. *Journal of Urology, 171*(2, Pt. 2), S19–S24.

Gann, P.H., & Giovannucci, E. (2004, September). Nutrition and prevention strategies for prostate cancer. In Prostate Cancer Foundation, *Report to the nation on prostate cancer 2004.* Retrieved February 26, 2008, from http://www.medscape.com/viewprogram/3447_pnt

Giovannucci, E., Ascherio, A., & Rimm, E.B. (1995). Intake of carotenoids and retinol in relation to prostate cancer risk. *Journal of the National Cancer Institute, 87*(23), 1767–1776.

Giovannucci, E., Liu, Y., Stampfer, M. J., & Willet, W.C. (2006). A prospective study of calcium intake and incident and fatal prostate cancer. *Cancer Epidemiology, Biomarkers and Prevention, 15*(2), 203–210.

Giovannucci, E., Rimm, E.B., Ascherio, A., Colditz, G.A., Spiegelman, D., Stampfer, M.J., et al. (1999). Smoking and risk of total and fatal prostate cancer in United States health care professionals. *Cancer Epidemiology, Biomarkers and Prevention, 8*(4, Pt. 1), 277–282.

Giovannucci, E., Rimm, E.B., Colditz, G.A., Stampfer, M.J., Ascherio, A., Chute, C.C., et al. (1993). A prospective study of dietary fat and risk of prostate cancer. *Journal of the National Cancer Institute, 85*(19), 1571–1579.

Giovannucci, E., Rimm, E.B., Liu, Y., Stampfer, M.J., & Willett, W.C. (2002). A prospective study of tomato products, lycopene, and prostate cancer risk. *Journal of the National Cancer Institute, 94*(5), 391–398.

Giovannucci, E., Rimm, E.B., Wolk, A., Ascherio, A., Stampfer, M.J., Colditz, G.A., et al. (1998). Calcium and fructose intake in relation to risk of prostate cancer. *Cancer Research, 58*(3), 442–447.

Gong, Z., Agalliu, I., Lin, D.W., Stanford, J.L., & Kristal, A.R. (2008). Cigarette smoking and prostate cancer-specific mortality following diagnosis in middle-aged men. *Cancer Causes and Control, 19*(1), 25–31.

Greene, K.L., Meng, M.V., Elkin, E.P., Cooperberg, M.R., Pasta, D.J., Kattan, M.W., et al. (2004). Validation of the Kattan preoperative nomogram for prostate cancer recurrence using a community based cohort: Results from Cancer of the Prostate Strategic Urological Research Endeavor (CaPSURE). *Journal of Urology, 171*(6, Pt. 1), 2255–2259.

Gronberg, H., Xu, J., Smith, J.R., Carpten, J.D., Isaacs, S.D., Freije, D., et al. (1997). Early age at diagnosis in families providing evidence of linkage to the hereditary prostate cancer locus (HPC1) on chromosome 1. *Cancer Research, 57*(21), 4707–4709.

Handayani, R., Rice, L., Cui, Y., Medrano, T.A., Samedi, V.G., Baker, H.V., et al. (2006). Soy isoflavones alter expression of genes associated with cancer progression, including interleukin-8, in androgen-independent PC-3 human prostate cancer cells. *Journal of Nutrition, 136*(1), 75–82.

Hayes, R.B., Ziegler, R.G., Gridley, G., Swanson, C., Greenberg, R.S., Swanson, G.M., et al. (1999). Dietary factors and risks for prostate cancer among blacks and whites in the United States. *Cancer Epidemiology, Biomarkers and Prevention, 8*(1), 25–34.

Heinonen, O.P., Albanes, D., Virtamo, J., Taylor, P.R., Huttunen, J.K., Hartman, A.M., et al. (1998). Prostate cancer and supplementation with alpha-tocopherol and beta-carotene: Incidence and mortality in a controlled trial. *Journal of the National Cancer Institute, 90*(6), 440–446.

Held-Warmkessel, J. (2005). Prostate cancer. In C.H. Yarbro, M.H. Frogge, & M. Goodman (Eds.), *Cancer nursing: Principles and practice* (6th ed., pp. 1552–1580). Sudbury, MA: Jones and Bartlett.

Hoffman, R.M., Blume, P., & Gilliland, F. (1998). Prostate-specific antigen testing practices and outcomes. *Journal of General Internal Medicine, 13*(2), 106–110.

Hsing, A.W., Tsao, L., & Devesa, S.S. (2000). International trends and patterns of prostate cancer incidence and mortality. *International Journal of Cancer, 85*(1), 60–67.

Hu, J.C., Elkin, E.P., Pasta, D.J., Lubeck, D.P., Kattan, M.W., Carroll, P.R., et al. (2004). Predicting quality of life after radical prostatectomy: Results from CaPSURE. *Journal of Urology, 171*(2, Pt. 1), 703–708.

Irvine, R.A., Ma, H., Yu, M.C., Ross, R.K., Stallcup, M.R., & Coetzee, G.A. (2000). Inhibition of p160-mediated coactivation with increasing androgen receptor polyglutamine length. *Human Molecular Genetics, 9*(2), 267–274.

Irvine, R.A., Yu, M.C., Ross, R.K., & Coetzee, G.A. (1995). The CAG and GGC microsatellites of the androgen receptor gene are in linkage disequilibrium in men with prostate cancer. *Cancer Research, 55*(9), 1937–1940.

Jemal, A., Siegel, R., Ward, E., Hao, Y., Xu, J., Murray, T., et al. (2008). Cancer statistics, 2008. *CA: A Cancer Journal for Clinicians, 58*(2), 71–96.

Johns, L.E., & Houlston, R.S. (2003). A systemic review and meta-analysis of familial prostate cancer risk. *BJU International, 91*(9), 789–794.

Jones, G.W., Mettlin, C., Murphy, G.P., Guinan, P., Herr, H.W., Hussey, D.H., et al. (1995). Patterns of care for carcinoma of the prostate gland: Results of a national survey of 1984 and 1990. *Journal of the American College of Surgeons, 180*(5), 545–554.

Kattan, M.W. (2007). Commentary: Should physicians use the updated Partin tables to predict pathologic stage in patients with prostate cancer? *Nature Clinical Practice: Urology, 4*(11), 593.

Kattan, M.W., Eastham, J.A., Stapleton, A.M., Wheeler, T.M., & Scardino, P.T. (1998). A preoperative nomogram for disease recurrence following radical prostatectomy for prostate cancer. *Journal of the National Cancer Institute, 90*(10), 766–771.

Klein, E.A., Thompson, I.M., Lippman, S.M., Goodman, P.J., Albanes, D., Taylor, P.R., et al. (2001). SELECT: The next prostate cancer prevention trial. Selenium and Vitamin E Cancer Prevention Trial. *Journal of Urology, 166*(4), 1311–1315.

Klein, E.A., Thompson, I.M., Lippman, S.M., Goodman, P.J., Albanes, D., Taylor, P.R., et al. (2003). SELECT: The Selenium and Vitamin E Cancer Prevention trial. *Urologic Oncology, 21*(1), 59–65, 145–151.

Kolonel, L.N., Hankin, J.H., Whittemore, A.S., Wu, A.H., Gallagher, R.P., Wilkins, L.R., et al. (2000). Vegetables, fruits, legumes and prostate cancer: A multiethnic case-control study. *Cancer Epidemiology, Biomarkers and Prevention, 9*(8), 795–804.

Kucuk, O., Sarkar, F.H., Sakr, W., Djuric, C., Pollack, M.N., Khachik, F., et al. (2001). Phase II randomized clinical trial of lycopene supplementation before radical prostatectomy. *Cancer Epidemiology, Biomarkers and Prevention, 10*(8), 861–868.

Kumar, N.B., Besterman-Dahan, L., Kang, J., Powsang, P., Xu, K., Allen, D., et al. (2008, February). *Lycopene in prostate cancer.* Abstract presented at the 2008 Genitourinary Cancers Symposium, San Francisco, CA. Retrieved March 28, 2008, from http://www.asco.org/ASCO/Abstracts+%26+Virtual+Meeting/Abstracts?&vmview=abst_detail_view&confID=54&abstractID=20547

Lam, J.S., Cheung, Y.K., Benson, M.C., & Goluboff, E.T. (2003). Comparison of the predictive accuracy of serum prostate specific antigen levels and prostate specific antigen density in the detection of prostate cancer in Hispanic-American and white men. *Journal of Urology, 170*(2, Pt. 1), 451–456.

Langeberg, W.J., Isaacs, W.B., & Stanford, J.L. (2007). Genetic etiology of hereditary prostate cancer. *Frontiers in Bioscience, 12,* 4101–4110.

Lee, M.M., Gomez, S.L., Chang, J.S., Wey, M., Wang, R.T., & Hsing, A.W. (2003). Soy and isoflavone consumption in relation to prostate cancer risk in China. *Cancer Epidemiology, Biomarkers and Prevention, 12*(7), 665–668.

Linehan, W.M., Zbar, B., Leach, F., Cordon-Cardo, C., & Isaacs, W. (2001). Molecular biology of genitourinary cancer. In V.T. DeVita Jr., S. Hellman, & S.A. Rosenberg (Eds.), *Cancer: Principles and practice of oncology* (6th ed., pp. 1343–1360). Philadelphia: Lippincott Williams & Wilkins.

Linn, M.M., Ball, R.A., & Maradiegue, A. (2007). Prostate-specific antigen screening: Friend or foe? *Urologic Nursing, 27*(6), 481–489.

Loeb, S., & Catalona, W.J. (2007). Prostate-specific antigen in clinical practice. *Cancer Letters, 249*(1), 30–39.

Loeb, S., Roehl, K.A., Yu, X., Han, M., & Catalona, W.J. (2007). Use of prostate-specific antigen velocity to follow up patients with isolated high-grade prostatic intraepithelial neoplasia on prostate biopsy. *Urology, 69*(1), 108–112.

Makarov, D.V., Trock, B.J., Humphreys, E.B., Mangold, L.A., Walsh, P.C., Epstein, J.I., et al. (2007). Updated nomogram to predict pathologic stage of prostate cancer given prostate-specific antigen level, clinical stage, and biopsy Gleason score (Partin tables) based on cases from 2000 to 2005. *Urology, 69*(6), 1095–1101.

Marcelli, M., Ittmann, M., Marian, S., Sutherland, R., Nigam, R., Murthy, L., et al. (2000). Androgen receptor mutations in prostate cancer. *Cancer Research, 60*(4), 944–949.

McDavid, K., Lee, J., Fulton, J.P., Tonita, J., & Thompson, T.D. (2004). Prostate cancer incidence and mortality rates and trends in the United States and Canada. *Public Health Report, 119*(2), 174–186.

McKee, J.M. (1994). Cues to action in prostate cancer screening. *Oncology Nursing Forum, 21*(7), 1171–1176.

Meiser, B., Cowan, R., Costello, A., Giles, G.G., Lindeman, G.J., & Gaff, C.L. (2007). Prostate cancer screening in men with a family history of prostate cancer: The role of partners in influencing men's screening uptake. *Urology, 70*(4), 738–742.

Menhert, A., Lehmann, C., Schulte, T., & Koch, U. (2007). Presence of symptoms distress and prostate cancer-related anxiety in patients at the beginning of cancer rehabilitation. *Onkologie, 30*(11), 551–556.

Mills, P.K., Beeson, W.L., Phillips, R.I., & Fraser, G.E. (1989). Cohort study of diet, lifestyle, and prostate cancer in Adventist men. *Cancer, 64*(3), 598–604.

Morgan, T.O., Jacobsen, S.J., McCarthy, W.F., Jacobson, D.J., McLeod, D.G., & Moul, J.W. (1996). Age-specific reference ranges for serum prostate-specific antigen in black men. *New England Journal of Medicine, 335*(5), 304–310.

Moul, J.W., Sesterhenn, I.A., Connelly, R.R., Douglas, T., Srivastava, S., Mostofi, F.K., et al. (1995). Prostate specific antigen values at the time of prostate cancer diagnosis in African-American men. *JAMA, 274*(16), 1277–1281.

National Cancer Institute. (2004). *Contents of the SEER cancer statistics review, 1975–2004.* Retrieved March 7, 2008, from http://seer.cancer.gov/csr/1975_2004/results_merged/sect_23_prostate.pdf

National Cancer Institute. (2008). *Clinical trials.* Retrieved January 20, 2008, from http://www.cancer.gov/clinicaltrials

National Comprehensive Cancer Network. (2007). *NCCN Clinical Practice Guidelines in Oncology™: Prostate cancer early detection* [v.2.2007]. Retrieved March 7, 2008, from http://www.nccn.org/professionals/physician_gls/PDF/prostate_detection.pdf

Nelson, W.G., DeMarzo, A.M., & Isaacs, W.B. (2003). Prostate cancer. *New England Journal of Medicine, 349*(4), 366–381.

Nilsen, T.I., Johnsen, R., & Vatten, L.J. (2000). Socio-economic and lifestyle factors associated with the risk of prostate cancer. *British Journal of Cancer, 82*(7), 1358–1363.

Oesterling, J.E. (1995). Using prostate-specific antigen to eliminate unnecessary diagnostic tests: Significant worldwide economic implications. *Urology, 46*(3, Suppl. A), 26–33.

Olson, M.C., Posniak, H.V., Fisher, S.G., Flisak, M.E., Salomon, C.G., Flanigan, R.C., et al. (1994). Directed and random biopsies of the prostate: Indications based on combined results of transrectal sonography and prostate-specific antigen density determinations. *American Journal of Roentgenology, 163*(6), 1407–1411.

Omenn, G.S., Goodman, G.E., Thornquist, M.D., Balmes, J., Cullen, M.R., Glass, A., et al. (1996). Risk factors for lung cancer and for intervention effects in CARET, the beta-Carotene and Retinol Efficacy Trial. *Journal of the National Cancer Institute, 88*(21), 1550–1559.

O'Rourke, M. (2005). Nursing care of the client with cancers of the urinary system. In J.K. Itano & K.N. Taoka (Eds.), *Core curriculum for oncology nursing* (4th ed., pp. 584–614). Philadelphia: Elsevier Saunders.

Pantuck, A.J., Leppert, J.T., Zomorodian, N., Aronson, W., Hong, J., Barnard, R.J., et al. (2006). Phase II study of pomegranate juice for men with rising prostate-specific antigen following surgery or radiation for prostate cancer. *Clinical Cancer Research, 12*(13), 4018–4026.

Pantuck, A.J., Zomorodian, N., Seeram, N., Rettig, M., Klatte, T., Heber, D., et al. (2008, February). *Long term follow up of pomegranate juice for men with prostate cancer and rising PSA shows durable improvement in PSA doubling time.* Abstract presented at the 2008 Genitourinary Cancers Symposium, San Francisco, CA. Retrieved March 28, 2008, from http://www.asco.org/ASCO/Abstracts+%26+Virtual+Meeting/Abstracts?&vmview=abst_detail_view&confID=54&abstractID=20241

Partin, A.W., Yoo, J., Carter, H.B., Pearson, J.D., Chan, D.W., Epstein, J.I., et al. (1993). The use of PSA clinical stage and Gleason score to predict pathologic stage in men with localized prostate cancer. *Journal of Urology, 150*(1), 110–114.

Pinsky, P.F., Andriole, G., Crawford, E.D., Chia, D., Kramer, B.S., Grubb, R., et al. (2007). Prostate-specific antigen velocity and prostate cancer Gleason grade and stage. *Cancer, 109*(8), 1689–1695.

Plaskon, L.A., Penson, D.F., Vaughan, T.L., & Stanford, J.L. (2003). Cigarette smoking and risk of prostate cancer in middle-aged men. *Cancer Epidemiology, Biomarkers and Prevention, 12*(7), 604–609.

Platz, E.A., Leitzmann, M.F., Rimm, E.B., Willet, W.C., & Giovannucci, E. (2004). Alcohol intake, drinking patterns, and risk of prostate cancer in large prospective cohort study. *American Journal of Epidemiology, 159*(5), 444–453.

Pound, C.R., Partin, A.W., Eisenberger, M.A., Chan, D.W., Pearson, J.D., & Walsh, P.C. (1999). Natural history of progression after PSA elevation following radical prostatectomy. *JAMA, 281*(17), 1591–1597.

Presti, J.C., Hovey, R., Bhargava, V., Carroll, P.R., & Shinohara, K. (1997). Prospective evaluation of prostate specific antigen and prostate specific antigen density in the detection of carcinoma of the prostate: Ethnic variations. *Journal of Urology, 157*(3), 907–911.

Price, D., Stein, B., Sieber, P., Tutrone, R., Bailen, J., Goluboff, E., et al. (2006). Toremifene for the prevention of prostate cancer in men with high grade prostatic intraepithelial neoplasia: Results of a double-blind placebo controlled, phase IIB clinical trial. *Journal of Urology, 176*(3), 965–970.

Putnam, S.D., Cerhan, J.R., Parker, A.S., Bianchi, G.D., Wallace, R.B., Cantor, K.P., et al. (2000). Lifestyle and anthropometric risk factors for prostate cancer in a cohort of Iowa men. *Annals of Epidemiology, 10*(6), 361–369.

Ramon, J.M., Bou, R., Romea, S., Alkiza, M.E., Jacas, M., Ribes, J., et al. (2000). Dietary intake and prostate cancer risk: A case control study in Spain. *Cancer Causes and Control, 11*(8), 679–685.

Rackley, J.D., Clark, P.E., & Hall, M.C. (2006). Complementary and alternative medicine for advanced prostate cancer. *Urologic Clinics of North America, 33*(2), 237–246.

Ries, L.A.G., Melbert, D., Krapcho, M., Mariotto, A., Miller, B.A., Feuer, E.J., et al. (Eds.). (2007). *SEER cancer statistics review, 1975–2004, National Cancer Institute.* Retrieved March 28, 2008, from http://seer.cancer.gov/csr/1975_2004

Rodriguez, C., McCullough, M.L., Mondul, A.M., Jacobs, E.J., Fakhrabadi-Shokoohi, D., Giovannucci, E.L., et al. (2003). Calcium dairy products and risk of prostate cancer in a prospective cohort of United States men. *Cancer Epidemiology, Biomarkers and Prevention, 12*(7), 597–603.

Rodriguez, C., Tatham, L.M., Thun, M.J., Calle, E.E., & Heath, C.W. (1997). Smoking and fatal prostate cancer in a large cohort of adult men. *American Journal of Epidemiology, 145*(5), 466–475.

Roobol, M.J., Grenabo, A., Schroder, F.H., & Hugosson, J. (2007). Interval cancers in prostate cancer screening: Comparing 2- and 4-year screening intervals in the European randomized study of screening for prostate cancer, Gothenburg and Rotterdam. *Journal of the National Cancer Institute, 99*(17), 1296–1303.

Saidi, O., Cordon-Cardo, C., & Costa, J. (2007). Technology insight: Will systems pathology replace the pathologist? *Nature Clinical Practice: Urology, 4*(1), 39–45.

Sanchez, M.A., Bowen, D.J., Hart, A., & Spigner, C. (2007). Factors influencing prostate cancer screening decisions among African American men. *Ethnicity and Disease, 17*(2), 374–380.

Schaid, D.J. (2004). The complex genetic epidemiology of prostate cancer. *Human Molecular Genetics, 13*(Special No. 1), R03–R121.

Schuurman, A.G., Goldbohm, R.A., & van den Brandt, P.A. (1999). A prospective cohort study on consumption of alcoholic beverages in relation to prostate cancer incidence (the Netherlands). *Cancer Causes and Control, 10*(6), 597–605.

Schuurman, A.G., van den Brandt, P.A., Dorant, E., Brants, H.A., & Goldbohm, R.A. (1999). Association of energy and fat intake with prostate carcinoma risk: Results from the Netherlands Cohort Study. *Cancer, 86*(6), 1019–1027.

Sesso, H., Paffenbarger, R., & Lee, I. (2001). Alcohol consumption and risk of prostate cancer: The Harvard Alumni Health Study. *International Journal of Epidemiology, 30*(4), 749–755.

Shimizu, H., Ross, R.K., Bernstein, L., Yatani, R., Henderson, B.E., & Mack, T.M. (1991). Cancers of the prostate and breast among Japanese and white immigrants in Los Angeles County. *British Journal of Cancer, 63*(6), 963–966.

Sim, H.G., & Cheng, C.W. (2005). Changing demography of prostate cancer in Asia. *European Journal of Cancer, 41*(6), 834–845.

Sirovich, B.E., Schwartz, L.M., & Woloshin, S. (2003). Screening men for prostate and colorectal cancer in the United States: Does practice reflect the evidence? *JAMA, 289*(11), 1414–1420.

Sofikerim, M., Eskicorapci, S., Oruc, O., & Ozen, H. (2007). Hormonal predictors of prostate cancer. *Urologia Internationalis, 79*(1), 13–18.

Spurgeon, S.E., Mongoue-Tchokote, S., Collins, L., Priest, R., Hsieh, Y.C., Peters, L.M., et al. (2007). Assessment of prostate-specific antigen doubling time in prediction of prostate cancer on needle biopsy. *Urology, 69*(5), 931–935.

Starr, S., Waldman, A.R., Tester, W., Kinsey, K.K., & Smith, D.T. (2002, November). *Awareness of prostate cancer in African American men and its influence on screening health behaviors* [Abstract No. 43734]. Poster presentation at the American Public Health Association Annual Meeting, Philadelphia, PA. Retrieved March 12, 2008, from http://apha.confex.com/apha/130am/techprogram/paper_43734.htm

Sun, J., Lange, E.M., Isaacs, S.D., Liu, W., Wiley, K.E., Lange, L., et al. (2008). Chromosome 8q24 risk variants in hereditary and non-hereditary prostate cancer patients. *Prostate, 68*(5), 489–497.

Sutcliffe, S., Giovannucci, E., Leitzmann, M.F., Rimm, E.B., Stampfer, M.J., Willet, W.C., et al. (2007). A prospective cohort study of red wine consumption and risk of prostate cancer. *International Journal of Cancer, 120*(7), 1529–1535.

Thompson, I.M., Ankerst, D., Chi, C., Goodman, P., Tangen, C., Lucia, M., et al. (2006). Assessing prostate cancer: Results from the prostate cancer prevention trial. *Journal of the National Cancer Institute, 98*(8), 529–534.

Thompson, I.M., Goodman, P.J., Tangen, C.M., Lucia, M.S., Miller, G.J., Ford, L.G., et al. (2003). The influence of finasteride on the development of prostate cancer. *New England Journal of Medicine, 349*(3), 215–224.

Thorpe, J.F., Jain, S., Marczylo, T.H., Gescher, A.J., Steward, W.P., & Mellon, J.K. (2007). A review of phase III clinical trials of prostate cancer chemoprevention. *Annals of the Royal College of Surgeons of England, 89*(3), 207–211.

U.S. Preventive Services Task Force. (2002a, December). *Screening for prostate cancer.* Recommendation statement. Retrieved September 22, 2008, from http://www.ahrq.gov/clinic/uspstf/08/prostate/prostaters.htm

U.S. Preventive Services Task Force. (2002b). Screening for prostate cancer: Recommendation and rationale. *Annals of Internal Medicine, 137*(11), 915–916.

Velicer, C.M., Kristal, A., & White, E. (2006). Alcohol use and the risk of prostate cancer: Results from the VITAL cohort study. *Nutrition and Cancer, 56*(1), 50–56.

Venkateswaran, V., Fleshner, N.E., & Klotz, L.H. (2004). Synergistic effect of vitamin E and selenium in human prostate cancer cell lines. *Prostate Cancer and Prostatic Diseases, 7*(1), 54–56.

Verhage, B.A.J., Baffoe Bonnic, A.B., Baglietto, L., Smith, D.S., Bailey-Wilson, J.E., Beaty, T.H., et al. (2001). Autosomal dominant inheritance of prostate cancer: A confirmatory study. *Urology, 57*(1), 97–101.

Villeneuve, P.J., Johnson, K.C., Krieger, N., & Mao, Y. (1999). Risk factors for prostate cancer: Results from the Canadian National Enhanced Cancer Surveillance System. Canadian Cancer Registries Epidemiology Research Group. *Cancer Causes and Control, 10*(5), 355–367.

Virtamo, J., Pietinen, P., Huttunen, J.K., Korhonen, P., Malila, N., Virtanen, M.J., et al. (2003). Incidence of cancer and mortality following alpha-tocopherol and beta-carotene supplementation: A post-intervention follow-up. *JAMA, 290*(4), 476–485.

Volk, R.J., Cantor, S.B., Cass, A.R., Spann, S.J., Weller, S.C., & Krahn, M.D. (2004). Preferences of husbands and wives for outcomes of prostate cancer screening and treatment. *Journal of General Internal Medicine, 19*(4), 339–348.

Waldman, A.R. (2006). Screening and early detection. In J. Held-Warmkessel (Ed.), *Contemporary issues in prostate cancer: A nursing perspective* (2nd ed., pp. 44–59). Sudbury, MA: Jones and Bartlett.

Walsh, P.C., & Partin, A.W. (1997). Family history facilitates the early diagnosis of prostate carcinoma. *Cancer, 80*(9), 1871–1874.

Weinrich, S.P., Boyd, M.D., Weinrich, M., Greene, F., Reynolds, W.A., & Metlin, C. (1998). Increasing prostate cancer screening in African-American men with peer-educator and client-navigator interventions. *Journal of Cancer Education, 13*(4), 213–219.

Whittemore, A.S., Kolonel, L.N., Wu, A.H., John, E.M., Gallagher, R.P., Howe, G.R., et al. (1995). Prostate cancer in relation to diet, physical activity, and body size in blacks, whites and Asians in the United States and Canada. *Journal of the National Cancer Institute, 87*(9), 652–661.

Wu, A.H., Whittemore, A.S., Kolonel, L.N., John, E.M., Gallagher, R.P., West, D.W., et al. (1995). Serum androgens and sex hormone-binding globulins in relation to lifestyle factors in older African-American, white, and Asian men in the United States and Canada. *Cancer Epidemiology, Biomarkers and Prevention, 4*(7), 735–741.

Yoshizawa, K., Willett, W.C., Morris, S.J., Stampfer, M.J., Spiegelman, D., Rimm, E.B., et al. (1998). Study of prediagnostic selenium level in toenails and the risk of advanced prostate cancer. *Journal of the National Cancer Institute, 90*(16), 1219–1224.

Zeegers, M., Jellema, A., & Ostrer, H. (2003). Empiric risk of prostate carcinoma for relatives of patients with prostate carcinoma: A meta-analysis. *Cancer, 97*(8), 1894–1903.

Zhou, J.R., Gugger, E.T., Tanaka, T., Guo, Y., Blackburn, G.L., & Clinton, S.K., et al. (1999). Soybeans phytochemicals inhibit the growth of transplantable human prostate carcinoma and tumor angiogenesis in mice. *Journal of Nutrition, 129*(9), 1628–1635.

CHAPTER 4

Treatment Modalities for Prostate Cancer

Marilyn L. Haas, PhD, RN, CNS, ANP-C, and Sarah Yenser Wood, RN, MSN, ANP, AOCNP®

Introduction

An estimated 186,320 men will be diagnosed with prostate cancer in 2008 (Jemal et al., 2008), and each of them have a number of treatment options from which to choose. These options include active surveillance (also known as watchful waiting or expectant management), surgery, radiation, or medical management of their disease. Treatment decisions are based on a number of complex factors, including the patient's physical status, tumor burden, and patient and physician preference. This chapter will examine current treatment options for prostate cancer and the rationale for their use.

Active Surveillance

Active surveillance of prostate cancer is an option for men with low-risk disease, which is defined as a T1–T2a tumor, a Gleason score (GS) between 2 and 6, and a prostate-specific antigen (PSA) level less than 10 ng/ml with any length of life expectancy. It also may be an option for men with moderate-risk disease, defined as a T2b–T2c tumor, a GS greater than 7, or a PSA level of 10–20 ng/ml with a life expectancy of 10 years or less (National Comprehensive Cancer Network [NCCN], 2007). In a study completed in Toronto, 299 men with low-risk (80%) to intermediate-risk (20%) prostate cancer were followed by active surveillance (Klotz, 2005). Men younger than age 70 were considered to be eligible for the trial if their PSA level was less than or equal to 10 and their GS was less than or equal to 6. Men older than age 70 were eligible for the trial if their PSA level was less than or equal to 15 and their GS was less than or equal to 7 (3 + 4). If the patient's PSA doubling time was less than two years (later changed to three years), repeat biopsy showed an increase in GS to 8 or higher (later changed to GS 7 (4 + 3)], or if the patient chose, delayed intervention was initiated as appropriate. Thirty-four percent of patients (N

= 101) came off of watchful waiting—3% for clinical signs of progression, 15% for PSA doubling time, 4% for increase in GS on repeat biopsy, and 12% because of patient choice (Klotz, 2005). Eighty-five percent of patients where alive at eight years, and only four patient deaths were related to prostate cancer (Klotz, 2006). These outcomes suggest that active surveillance may be an appropriate alternative for some men with prostate cancer.

By choosing active surveillance, men are able to avoid side effects commonly associated with more aggressive treatment options, such as sexual dysfunction and urinary and bowel dysfunction (Bremner, Chong, Tomlinson, Alibhai, & Krahn, 2007). Men participating in active surveillance can still maintain a similar quality of life and 10-year survival rates when compared to those who underwent prostatectomy or radiation as primary treatment (Choo et al., 2002). It also gives men the opportunity to avoid treatment altogether if they have a slow-growing tumor. Unfortunately, if disease progression is present during this time, the chance for cure may be missed, leading to the development of metastatic disease and resulting in the need for second-line or salvage treatment. Figure 4-1 lists the principles of active surveillance (i.e., expectant management) as put forth by NCCN (2007).

Patients choosing expectant management should be followed with a digital rectal examination (DRE) and PSA testing every 6 months if they are expected to live 10 years or more and every 6–12 months if they are expected to live less than 10 years. Additionally, patients should have repeat needle biopsies 6–18 months after diagnosis, depending on the number of cores sampled during the original biopsy. Some controversy exists regarding the definition of disease progression in this population. NCCN (2007) defined prostate cancer disease progression as a PSA doubling time of less than three years, an increase in the number of positive biopsy cores, or an increase in the GS. Alternatively, a study completed by Choo et al. (2002) defined progression as a PSA doubling time of less than two years, an increase in the GS on repeat biopsy, or clinical progression. Once progression occurs, treatment with

Figure 4-1. National Comprehensive Cancer Network Principles of Expectant Management

- Expectant management involves actively monitoring the course of disease with the expectation to intervene if the cancer progresses.
- Patients with clinically localized cancers who are candidates for definitive treatment and choose expectant management should have regular follow up:
  - DRE and PSA every 6 months for life expectancy ≥ 10 years and every 6–12 months for life expectancy < 10 years
  - Needle biopsy of the prostate may be repeated within 6 months of diagnosis if initial biopsy was < 10 cores or assessment discordant (e.g., palpable tumor contralateral to side of positive biopsy)
  - Needle biopsy may be performed within 18 months if > 10 cores obtained initially, then periodically.
- Cancer progression may have occurred if:
  - Primary Gleason grade 4 or 5 cancer is found upon repeat prostate biopsy
  - Prostate cancer is found in a greater number of prostate biopsies or occupies a greater extent of prostate biopsies
  - PSA doubling time < 3 years or PSA velocity > 0.75.
- A repeat prostate biopsy is indicated for signs of disease progression by exam or PSA.
- Advantages of expectant management:
  - Avoid possible side effects of definitive therapy that may be unnecessary
  - Quality of life/normal activities retained
  - Risk of unnecessary treatment of small, indolent cancers is reduced.
- Disadvantages of expectant management:
  - Chance of missed opportunity for cure
  - Risk of progression and/or metastases
  - Subsequent treatment may be more intense with increased side effects
  - Nerve sparing may be more difficult, which may reduce chance of potency preservation after surgery
  - Increased anxiety
  - Requires frequent medical exams and periodic biopsies
  - Uncertain long term natural history of prostate cancer.

DRE—digital rectal examination; PSA—prostate-specific antigen

Note. Reproduced with permission from The *NCCN 2.2007 Prostate Cancer Clinical Practice Guidelines in Oncology.* © National Comprehensive Cancer Network, 2007. Available at http://www.nccn.org. Accessed January 29, 2008. To view the most recent and complete version of the guideline, go online to www.nccn.org.

These Guidelines are a work in progress that will be refined as often as new significant data become available.

The NCCN Guidelines are a statement of consensus of its authors regarding their views of currently accepted approaches to treatment. Any clinician seeking to apply or consult any NCCN guideline is expected to use independent medical judgment in the context of individual clinical circumstances to determine any patient's care or treatment. The National Comprehensive Cancer Network makes no warranties of any kind whatsoever regarding their content, use or application and disclaims any responsibility for their application or use in any way.

These Guidelines are copyrighted by the National Comprehensive Cancer Network. All rights reserved. These Guidelines and illustrations herein may not be reproduced in any form for any purpose without the express written permission of the NCCN.

radiation, surgery, or hormonal therapy should be initiated, regardless of which definition is used.

The challenge of active surveillance is determining which patients will benefit from such a treatment approach versus undergoing definitive therapy. Only 2%–3% of men who develop prostate cancer actually die of the disease (Kirby, Christmas, & Brawer, 2001). Active surveillance should be a decision arrived at by the patient and the practitioner with input from the patient's significant others. Reasons for choosing active surveillance may include patient reluctance or fear of surgical intervention, incidence of treatment-related morbidity, advanced age, and presence of comorbid conditions. Although more popular in Europe, active surveillance will likely not gain widespread recognition and support in the absence of strong supportive evidence from large, prospective randomized trials (Held-Warmkessel, 2005).

Hormonal Manipulation

Hormonal manipulation, or hormonal therapy, has long been an important staple in the treatment of prostate cancer. It is used in the adjuvant and salvage clinical settings, with current trends using hormone manipulation in earlier stages of disease. Castration is the first-line treatment for metastatic prostate cancer and can be achieved surgically or medically, both of which are equally effective methods. Neoadjuvant hormonal therapy before radical prostatectomy is strongly discouraged (NCCN, 2007). Some prostate cancer cells thrive in an androgen-rich environment. Malignant prostate tissue can consist of androgen-dependent, androgen-sensitive, and androgen-independent cells (Isaacs et al., 1992). When androgen sources are eliminated, androgen-dependent cells cease to exist, and androgen-sensitive cells no longer divide (Martikainen, Kyprianou, Tucker, & Isaacs, 1991). The testes produce most of the androgen, and secretion is dependent on luteinizing hormone-releasing hormone (LHRH). Reducing the circulating serum androgen level in a patient with prostate cancer is preferred if metastatic disease is present at the time of diagnosis, if a rising PSA level exists after surgery or radiation therapy, or if the patient is unable to undergo surgery or radiation or refuses such treatment, or in conjunction with adjuvant radiation therapy (NCCN). See Figure 4-2 for principles of hormonal therapy (i.e., androgen deprivation therapy [ADT]) as put forth by NCCN.

Surgical Castration

A bilateral orchiectomy is an outpatient surgical procedure in which the testes are removed, thereby decreasing testosterone production. Following orchiectomy, testosterone production decreases by 90%–95% (Schroder, 1998), with the remaining production coming from the adrenal glands. Orchiectomy is a relatively simple procedure and usually is

---

Figure 4-2. National Comprehensive Cancer Network Principles of Hormonal Therapy (Androgen Deprivation Therapy [ADT])

Neoadjuvant ADT for Clinically Localized Disease
- Neoadjuvant ADT for radical prostatectomy is strongly discouraged.
- Giving ADT before, during and/or after radiation prolongs survival in selected radiation managed patients.
- Adjuvant ADT given after completion of primary treatment is not a standard treatment at this time with the exception of selected high-risk patients treated with radiation therapy.
- In the largest randomized trial to date using antiandrogen bicalutamide alone at high dose (150 mg), there were indications of a delay in recurrence of disease but no improvement in survival. Longer follow-up is needed.
- In one randomized trial, immediate and continuous use of ADT in men with positive nodes following radical prostatectomy resulted in significantly improved overall survival compared to men who received delayed ADT. Therefore, such patients should be considered for immediate ADT.

Timing of ADT for Advanced Disease (PSA recurrence or metastatic disease)
- The timing of ADT for patients whose only evidence of cancer is a rising PSA is influenced by PSA velocity, patient anxiety, and the short and long term side effects of ADT.
- A significant proportion of these patients will ultimately die of their disease; their prognosis is best approximated by the absolute level of PSA, the rate of change in the PSA level (PSA "doubling time"), and the initial stage, grade, and PSA level at the time of definitive therapy.
- Earlier ADT may be better than delayed ADT, although the definitions of early and late (what level of PSA) are controversial. Since the benefit of early ADT is not clear, treatment should be individualized until definitive studies are done. Patients with a short PSA doubling time (rapid PSA velocity) and an otherwise long life expectancy should be encouraged to consider ADT earlier, unless they regard the side effects as unacceptable.
- Treatment should begin immediately in the presence of tumor-related symptoms or overt metastases (category 1). Earlier ADT will delay the appearance of symptoms and of metastases, but it is not clear whether earlier ADT will prolong survival. The complications of long term ADT have not been adequately documented.

Optimal ADT
- LHRH agonist (medical castration) and bilateral orchiectomy (surgical castration) are equally effective.
- Combined androgen blockade (medical or surgical castration combined with an antiandrogen) provides no proven benefit over castration alone in patients with metastatic disease.
- Antiandrogen therapy should precede or be co-administered with LHRH agonist and be continued in combination for at least 7 days for patients with overt metastases who are at risk of developing symptoms associated with the flare in testosterone with initial LHRH agonist alone.
- Antiandrogen monotherapy appears to be less effective than medical or surgical castration and should not be recommended. The side effects are different but overall less tolerable.
- No clinical data support the use of triple androgen blockade (finasteride or dutasteride with combined androgen blockade).
- Intermittent androgen deprivation therapy is a widely used approach to reduce side effects, but the long-term efficacy remains unproven.
- Patients who do not achieve adequate suppression of serum testosterone (less than 50 ng/ml) with medical or surgical castration can be considered for additional hormonal manipulations (with estrogen, antiandrogens, or steroids), although the clinical benefit is not clear.

Secondary Hormonal Therapy
- The androgen receptor remains active in patients whose prostate cancer has recurred during androgen deprivation therapy (castration-recurrent prostate cancer); thus ADT should be continued.
- A variety of strategies can be employed if initial ADT has failed which may afford clinical benefit, including antiandrogen withdrawal, and administration of antiandrogens, ketoconazole, or estrogens; however, none of these has yet been demonstrated to prolong survival in randomized clinical trials.

Monitor/Surveillance
- Patients being treated with either medical or surgical castration are at risk for having or developing osteoporosis. A baseline bone mineral density study should be considered in this group of patients, especially if long term ADT is planned.
- Supplementation with calcium (500 mg daily) and vitamin D (400 IU) is recommended for all men on long-term ADT.
- Men who are osteopenic/osteoporotic should be strongly considered for bisphosphonate therapy with zoledronic acid, pamidronate, alendronate, raloxifene, or toremifene.

LHRH—luteinizing hormone-releasing hormone; PSA—prostate-specific antigen

Note. Reproduced with permission from *The NCCN 2.2007 Prostate Cancer Clinical Practice Guidelines in Oncology.* © National Comprehensive Cancer Network, 2007. Available at http://www.nccn.org. Accessed January 29, 2008. To view the most recent and complete version of the guideline, go online to www.nccn.org.

These Guidelines are a work in progress that will be refined as often as new significant data become available.
The NCCN Guidelines are a statement of consensus of its authors regarding their views of currently accepted approaches to treatment. Any clinician seeking to apply or consult any NCCN guideline is expected to use independent medical judgment in the context of individual clinical circumstances to determine any patient's care or treatment. The National Comprehensive Cancer Network makes no warranties of any kind whatsoever regarding their content, use or application and disclaims any responsibility for their application or use in any way.

These Guidelines are copyrighted by the National Comprehensive Cancer Network. All rights reserved. These Guidelines and illustrations herein may not be reproduced in any form for any purpose without the express written permission of the NCCN.

less expensive than medical castration. However, it often is not the treatment choice, as orchiectomy and its associated side effects are permanent, and the resultant body image issues are not favorable (Chon, Jacobs, & Naslund, 2000). If a man does choose to undergo orchiectomy, prosthetic testicles that look and feel similar to one's original anatomy can be surgically inserted into the scrotum.

Medical Castration

LHRH, released by the hypothalamus, is targeted by LHRH agonists to suppress testosterone production by inhibiting gonadotropin. LHRH agonists initially increase the production of testosterone resulting in a surge or a "flare" response. During a testosterone surge response, which may last for several days, malignant prostate cells could thrive. Additionally, symptoms such as bone pain and urinary outlet problems may increase. To prevent such a surge, patients are prescribed antiandrogens for at least seven days prior to initiating treatment with an LHRH agonist or concurrently for seven days. Some physicians continue both medications until PSA elevation occurs. The results have varied when using combined hormonal therapy from no significant survival benefit to a seven-month survival benefit (Moul, 2000).

Administration of a newer class of medications known as LHRH antagonists also results in medical castration but does not cause a surge of testosterone. LHRH antagonists work by blocking luteinizing hormone and follicle-stimulating hormone production and may be initiated without antiandrogen use.

LHRH agonists and antagonists are available in subcutaneous injections or implants and intramuscular injections, and administration schedules vary (see Table 4-1). The frequency of injection varies, and each allows patients the opportunity to pursue intermittent hormonal therapy if indicated.

Hormonal therapies also can be used in combination with both radiation and surgery. Multiple clinical trials have been performed using combined androgen blockade or LHRH agonists alone prior to, during, or after radiation therapy (European Organisation for Research and Treatment of Cancer study 22863, Radiation Therapy Oncology Group [RTOG] trial 85–31, RTOG trial 86–10, Trans-Tasman Radiation Oncology Group trial 96–01, RTOG protocol 92–02, and RTOG 94–13). All of these studies showed that the addition of hormonal therapy neoadjuvantly, adjuvantly, or concurrently to radiation resulted in improved survival or local control (Bolla, Descotes, Artignan, & Fourneret, 2007). An Eastern Cooperative Oncology Group clinical trial completed by Messing et al. (2006) randomized 100 men post-prostatectomy with confirmed lymph node metastasis, but no distant metastasis, to immediate treatment with medical or surgical castration (patient choice) or watchful waiting until evidence of clinical recurrence. These men were followed for survival. Those who received immediate hormonal treatment were found to have a survival advantage over those who received delayed treatment (Messing et al.). Using medical castration is not recommended prior to surgery, as no benefit has been established for improvement in survival, and some studies have shown that the use of neoadjuvant medical castration has made surgery more difficult (Pu, Wang, Wu, & Wang, 2007).

Intermittent hormonal therapy is used in men with prostate cancer who do not have metastatic disease to help to decrease the side effects of hormonal therapy, such as loss of libido, loss of bone density, muscle wasting, weight gain, and cardiac issues. Intermittent therapy also may be used to lengthen the time until the prostate cancer is able to grow without the presence of testosterone (McLeod, 2003). When this type of growth occurs, the disease becomes androgen-independent or hormone-refractory prostate cancer (HRPC). The long-term benefits of intermittent hormonal therapy are unknown and are being evaluated by clinical trials (Moul, 2000). Bruchovsky, Klotz, Crook, and Goldenberg (2007) examined intermittent hormonal manipulation in a phase II trial for men with recurrent prostate cancer following radiation therapy. The researchers suggested that the length of the off-treatment interval during cyclic hormonal manipulation was inversely related to baseline and nadir levels of serum PSA.

When prostate cancer no longer responds to hormonal therapy alone, secondary hormonal options or chemotherapy may be used (NCCN, 2007). Secondary hormonal options consist of three categories: antiandrogens, estrogens, and adrenal suppressive agents (see Table 4-2). These agents are used in patients with no metastasis, those with limited metastasis with no symptoms, or those who prefer to delay treatment with chemotherapy. Antiandrogens such as flutamide, bicalutamide, and nilutamide are medications that competitively bind to androgen receptor sites in the prostate cancer tissue, thus preventing the binding of testosterone and causing the cell growth to slow or stop and resulting in a reduction of PSA. Antiandrogens can be continued until PSA elevation occurs. When antiandrogens are discontinued, a resulting reduction in PSA can occur. This reduction is considered part of a "withdrawal effect." Further hormonal manipulation usually is held until PSA values begin to rise.

Bicalutamide 150 mg daily also has been studied versus placebo given concurrently with radiation, watchful waiting, or surgery for two years or until disease progression. In a randomized, double-blind study of 8,113 men with localized or locally advanced prostate cancer, the addition of bicalutamide demonstrated a significant survival advantage, reducing the risk of death by 35% (McLeod, Iversen, et al., 2006). Although these results are quite good, most of the survival benefit occurred in those with locally advanced disease rather than those with localized disease. As a result, bicalutamide is thought to be unnecessary in this population (McLeod, See, et al., 2006).

Estrogens are not frequently used in prostate cancer, in part because of their potential cardiovascular side effects,

Table 4-1. Luteinizing Hormone-Releasing Hormone (LHRH) Agonists and Antagonists

Medication	Means of Administration	Administration Schedule	Nursing Considerations
LHRH Agonists			
Goserelin acetate implant (Zoladex®, AstraZeneca Pharmaceuticals)	Subcutaneous (SC) implant to abdomen	Every 28 days or 3 months	Numb area for injection prior to injection.
Histrelin implant (Vantas®, Indevus Pharmaceuticals, Inc.)	SC implant to inner upper arm	Every 12 months	Will be inserted in an outpatient procedure. May require sutures.
Leuprolide acetate (Eligard®, QLT USA, Inc.)	Deep intramuscular (IM)	Every 1, 3, 4, or 6 months	Some formulations may contain benzyl alcohol and mannitol. Verify contents along with patient allergies prior to administration. Rotate injection sites. Mix well prior to administration.
Leuprolide acetate (Lupron®, TAP Pharmaceuticals Inc.)	IM	Every 1, 3, or 4 months	See above.
Leuprolide acetate implant (Viadur®, Bayer Pharmaceuticals Corp.)	SC implant to inner upper arm	Every 12 months	Will be inserted in an outpatient procedure. May require sutures.
LHRH Antagonist			
Abarelix (Plenaxis®, Praecis Pharmaceuticals)	Deep IM	Given on days 1, 15, 29 and then every 4 weeks	Monitor testosterone levels.

Note. Based on information from Clinical Pharmacology, 2008.

including deep vein thrombosis (DVT) and heart disease. However, they can be of benefit to patients who are unwilling or unable to undergo treatment with chemotherapy. A common estrogen used in prostate cancer, diethylstilbestrol (or DES) is no longer manufactured in the United States but is available at compounding pharmacies. In areas where compounding pharmacies are not available, some practitioners may prescribe Premarin® (Wyeth Pharmaceuticals). In clinical trials, it had a response rate of 20%–25% depending on the dose (Pomerantz et al., 2007). DVT and pulmonary embolus can be minimized by combining estrogen therapies with a prophylactic dose of warfarin. Gynecomastia (breast enlargement) and tenderness, also side effects of estrogen therapy, can be minimized with prophylactic breast irradiation. Radiation dosage typically ranges between 12–15 gray (Gy) given over three to four fractions (treatments) (Serber, Brady, Zhang, & Hoppe, 2004).

Ketoconazole is an adrenal suppressive agent approved by the U.S. Food and Drug Administration (FDA) for the treatment of fungal infections. Ketoconazole has a side effect of suppressing adrenal gland function, which is responsible for some testosterone production. Thus, circulating testosterone levels decrease, along with PSA levels. In one study, 28.3% of patients on low-dose ketoconazole (200 mg PO TID) had a PSA decline of greater than 50% (Nakabayashi et al., 2006). This was a retrospective study, and those who experienced a

rise in PSA typically were then given high-dose therapy (400 mg PO TID). Patients who had initially responded to low-dose therapy responded longer (2.9 months compared to 1.3 months) on high-dose therapy than those who did not respond to initial low-dose treatment. Patients who had received less ADT responded longer as well (4.1 months in patients who had received < 27.7 months of ADT versus 2.8 months in those who had been treated with ADT for > 27.7 months). Both low-dose and high-dose ketoconazole require the addition of a corticosteroid to the treatment regimen as cortisol secretion, a normal adrenal function, is decreased as well.

Bisphosphonate Therapy

Bisphosphonates can be used to prevent fracture in patients with osteoporosis caused by ADT and in patients with bone metastasis. Men being treated with ADT were randomized to either alendronate 70 mg weekly or placebo. Both groups received calcium 500 mg with vitamin D 200 units BID. The bone mineral density of the spine and hip increased significantly in the alendronate arm compared to the placebo group. Studies using raloxifene, pamidronate, and zoledronic acid also have shown some improvement in bone loss related to ADT (Greenspan, Nelson, Trump, & Resnick, 2007). In a study completed by Saad et al. (2002), men with prostate cancer and bone metastasis were

Table 4-2. Secondary Hormonal Options

Medication	Means of Administration	Administration Schedule	Nursing Considerations
Pure Antiandrogens			
Bicalutamide	50–150 mg PO	Daily	Monitor liver function tests (LFTs).
Flutamide	125 mg PO	2 tabs TID	Monitor LFTs.
Nilutamide	150–300 mg PO	300 mg daily for first 30 days, and then 150 mg daily	Monitor LFTs.
Estrogens/Progestins			
Conjugated estrogens	1.25–2.5 mg PO	Daily	Use with caution if soy allergy is present. Monitor for signs of DVT and PE. Consider prophylactic warfarin.
Diethylstilbestrol	1–3 mg PO	Daily	Available only through compounding pharmacies. Administer with warfarin. Monitor for signs of deep vein thrombosis (DVT) and pulmonary embolism (PE).
Megestrol acetate	40 mg PO	2–4 times daily	Monitor for signs of DVT and PE. Consider prophylactic warfarin.
Adrenal Suppressives			
Corticosteroids	Prednisone 7.5–10 mg PO or equivalent doses in other corticosteroids	Daily	Improves quality of life (Lam et al., 2006)
Ketoconazole	200–400 mg PO	TID	Give with hydrocortisone. Monitor LFTs.

Note. Based on information from Clinical Pharmacology, 2008.

randomized to either zoledronic acid (Zometa®, Novartis Pharmaceuticals Corp.) 4 mg IV every three weeks, Zometa 8 mg IV every three weeks (later dose was reduced to 4 mg because of safety concerns related to renal function), or placebo every three weeks. A significant reduction in skeletal-related events, an increase in length of time to first skeletal event, and a decrease in skeletal morbidity occurred. The 8 mg group was inferior to the 4 mg group and showed no statistically significant difference over the placebo group (Saad et al.). Studies are ongoing with other bisphosphonates in this clinical setting. Patients who are going to be treated with bisphosphonates should have a dental evaluation before initiation of therapy. Any necessary dental work should be completed and fully healed prior to starting therapy. While on treatment with bisphosphonates, patients should see their dentists regularly and inform them of the medications they are taking. A serious side effect known as osteonecrosis of the jaw can occur in 1%–10% of patients with cancer who are receiving bisphosphonates when tooth extraction or any extensive dental work is completed (Khosla et al., 2007).

Surgical Treatment

Transurethral Resection of the Prostate Gland

Transurethral resection of the prostate gland (TURP) frequently is performed to relieve urinary outlet obstruction symptoms from hypertrophy of the prostate gland or from the presence of a prostate tumor pressing against the gland itself. In most cases, benign prostatic hypertrophy is treated with medication or a TURP procedure. Incidental finding of prostate cancer may result following a TURP, but it is not the preferred method of diagnosis. TURP used in the setting of known prostate cancer is designed to alleviate symptoms from bladder outlet obstruction, including urinary urgency, frequency, difficulty or inability to void, urinary retention, overflow urinary incontinence, and lower abdominal pain. TURP is not performed with the intent to cure prostate cancer and usually is reserved for men older than 70 years of age with a life expectancy of less than 10 years (Berry, 2004; Frydenberg & Oesterling, 1997; Mason, 2006).

Three main options are available to men who choose surgical intervention as definitive treatment for prostate cancer: open radical prostatectomy, laparoscopic radical prostatectomy (LRP), and robot-assisted laparoscopic radical prostatectomy (RLRP). With the advent of PSA screening and early detection, the number of radical prostatectomies has increased (Pirtsvholaishvili, Hrebinko, & Nelson, 2001). Radical prostatectomy usually is performed when the tumor is localized (T1 or T2), life expectancy is greater than 10 years, and little to no significant comorbidities exist (NCCN, 2007). A radical prostatectomy consists of removal of the prostate, surrounding tissues, and seminal vesicles. Surgeons who perform a high number of radical prostatectomies in high-volume centers tend to provide better outcomes

(NCCN). Figure 4-3 lists the principles of surgery as put forth by NCCN.

Radical Perineal Prostatectomy

This open technique is performed through an incision in the perineum. This approach has been associated with decreased complications postoperatively in patients with pulmonary disease, decreased blood loss, and ease of performing the vesicourethral anastomosis as a result of improved visibility of the operative site (Mason, 2006). The hospital stay also may be shorter. Although this approach has its advantages, it is limited by increased erectile dysfunction and rectal injury, and a pelvic lymph node

---

Figure 4-3. National Comprehensive Cancer Network Principles of Surgery

Pelvic Lymph Node Dissection (PLND):
- An extended PLND includes removal of all node-bearing tissue from an area bounded by the external iliac vein anteriorly, the pelvic sidewall laterally, the bladder wall medially, the floor of the pelvis posteriorly, Cooper's ligament distally, and the internal iliac artery proximally.
- A limited PLND includes removal of all node-bearing tissue from an area bounded by the external iliac vein anteriorly, the pelvic sidewall laterally, the bladder wall medially, the obturator nerve posteriorly, Cooper's ligament distally, and internal iliac vein proximally.
- An extended PLND will discover metastases approximately twice as often as a limited PLND. Extended PLND provides more complete staging and may cure some men with microscopic metastases.
- Dissection of nodes anterior and lateral to the external iliac vessels is associated with an increased risk of lymphedema and is discouraged. Extended PLND compared to limited PLND increases the risk of lymphedema after external beam radiation therapy. In addition, an extra peritoneal dissection is preferred if EBRT is anticipated.
- A PLND can be excluded in patients with < 7% predicated probability of nodal metastases by nomograms, although some patients with lymph node metastases will be missed.
- PLND can be performed using an open, laparoscopic or robotic technique.
- An extra peritoneal dissection is preferred if EBRT is anticipated.

Radical Prostatectomy (RP):
- RP is appropriate therapy for any patient with clinically localized prostate cancer that can be completely excised surgically, who has a life expectancy of 10 years or more and no serious co-morbid conditions that would contraindicate an elective operation.
- High volume surgeons in high volume centers generally provide better outcomes.
- Laparoscopic and robot-assisted radical prostatectomy are used commonly. In experienced hands, the results of these approaches appear comparable to open surgical approaches.
- Blood loss can be substantial with radical prostatectomy but can be reduced by careful control of periprostatic vessels.
- Urinary incontinence can be reduced by preservation of urethral length beyond the apex of the prostate and avoiding damage to the distal sphincter mechanism. Bladder neck preservation may decrease the risk of incontinence. Anastomotic strictures increase the risk of long-term incontinence.
- Recovery of erectile function is directly related to the degree of preservation of the cavernous nerves. Replacement of resected nerves with nerve grafts is investigational. Early restoration of erections may improve late recovery.
- Salvage radical prostatectomy is an option for highly selected patients with local recurrence after EBRT, brachytherapy, or cryotherapy in the absence of metastases, but the morbidity (incontinence, loss of erection, anastomotic stricture) is high.

EBRT—external beam radiation therapy

Note. Reproduced with permission from *The NCCN 2.2007 Prostate Cancer Clinical Practice Guidelines in Oncology.* © National Comprehensive Cancer Network, 2007. Available at http://www.nccn.org. Accessed January 29, 2008. To view the most recent and complete version of the guideline, go online to www.nccn.org.

These Guidelines are a work in progress that will be refined as often as new significant data become available.
The NCCN Guidelines are a statement of consensus of its authors regarding their views of currently accepted approaches to treatment. Any clinician seeking to apply or consult any NCCN guideline is expected to use independent medical judgment in the context of individual clinical circumstances to determine any patient's care or treatment. The National Comprehensive Cancer Network makes no warranties of any kind whatsoever regarding their content, use or application and disclaims any responsibility for their application or use in any way.

These Guidelines are copyrighted by the National Comprehensive Cancer Network. All rights reserved. These Guidelines and illustrations herein may not be reproduced in any form for any purpose without the express written permission of the NCCN.

dissection (PLND) must be completed through a different incision.

Radical Retropubic Prostatectomy

Radical retropubic prostatectomy is a commonly used open technique performed through an incision in the lower abdomen from the umbilicus to the pubis. This technique allows for a PLND to be completed through the same incision and also provides an opportunity for nerve-sparing surgery if the cancer is not too extensive. Sparing the nerves often preserves erectile function (Mason, 2006).

Salvage Radical Prostatectomy

This approach may be used when patients have a local recurrence without metastases after external beam radiation therapy (EBRT), brachytherapy, or cryotherapy. This surgery is likely to result in more morbidity than if surgery were completed first, as it can cause a change in blood flow as well as an increase in scarring from the previous treatments. Urinary incontinence and erectile dysfunction are likely to occur in patients who undergo this procedure (Mason, 2006).

Minimally Invasive Radical Prostatectomy

With the advent of new technology has come the refinement of minimally invasive and laparoscopic surgical techniques. LRP was pioneered in the mid-1990s, and its popularity has grown as a result of advanced technology and patient preference. Decreased postsurgical healing time is the primary advantage to choosing LRP or RLRP. These minimally invasive surgical techniques have smaller incisions and typically allow for an easier postoperative convalescent period.

Although a surgeon's experience is more important than the approach, the use of the robot is thought to improve the precision and accuracy over the conventional laparoscopic approach (Herrmann et al., 2007). A surgeon's learning curve for mastering RLRP has been rated at 50 or more procedures (Cathelineau, Arroyo, Rozet, Baumert, & Vallancien, 2004). The use of robotic systems assists surgeons by enhancing dexterity and reducing tremors (Lanfranco, Castellanos, Desai, & Meyers, 2004). Intraoperative complications are uncommon but include ureter and bowel injuries and intra-abdominal urinary leakage (Bollens et al., 2002). A nerve-sparing approach can be utilized during RLRP, which may result in lower rates of erectile dysfunction, urinary incontinence, and disease recurrence when compared to the open procedure. Currently, however, outcomes and side effect profiles are equivalent, and current trials are ongoing to determine whether RLRP yields improved outcomes (Borden & Kozlowski, 2006).

Lymph Node Dissection

In addition to prostatectomy, some men may require a pelvic lymph node dissection. Lymph node dissections typically are completed in men thought to have high-risk disease defined as a PSA greater than 10 ng/ml and a total GS of greater than 6, although this remains at the surgeon's discretion (Dhar, Burkhard, & Studer, 2007). Pelvic lymph node dissection can be excluded in patients with less than 7% predicted probability of nodal metastases by nomogram (NCCN, 2007). Not only is the decision to complete a lymph node dissection not standard, but the extent of the dissection also varies widely among surgeons. A minimal dissection removes the lymph nodes in the obturator fossa; a standard dissection removes those in the obturator fossa and in the external iliac chain; and an extended dissection removes those in the obturator fossa and those in the external, internal, and common iliac chains (Dhar et al.). The minimal dissection is thought to miss about 50% of all positive nodes, as two-thirds of patients with positive lymph nodes will have positive internal iliac nodes, which are not sampled in a limited dissection (Dhar et al.). In patients with a low volume of lymph node metastasis, questions exist as to whether lymph node dissection confers any therapeutic value, which is why most surgeons agree that low-risk patients should not undergo dissections (Sivalingam, Oxley, Probert, Stolzenburg, & Schwaibold, 2007). If lymphadenectomy is performed, at least 20 lymph nodes are needed to show adequate staging. This may prove to be technically difficult, as identifying lymph nodes in the adipose tissue of the pelvic area is quite challenging (Sivalingam et al.). In addition, the potential for lower-extremity lymphedema, especially following EBRT, further discourages many patients and surgeons from opting for this relatively low-yield intervention.

Cryosurgery

Another type of surgical intervention for prostate cancer involves freezing the gland. Developed in 1990, cryosurgery consists of insertion of a transperineal cryoprobe into the prostate via transrectal ultrasound guidance (Moul, 2000). The probe uses super-cooled liquid nitrogen, argon gas, or helium to freeze the prostate gland to a temperature of approximately $-100°F$ to $-200°F$ for 5–10 minutes. Cryosurgery is indicated for patients with localized high risk T1–T3 disease for which prostatectomy is contraindicated because of comorbidities or patient choice. It also can be used to debulk large primary prostate tumors for patients with or without metastatic disease (De La Taille et al., 2000). Side effects of cryosurgery include urinary incontinence, erectile dysfunction, perineal or scrotal pain, and urethral tissue sloughing resulting in dysuria and hematuria. The placement of a urethral warming catheter decreases the incidence of urinary incontinence and significantly decreases the incidence of urethral tissue sloughing. Clinical trials examining the appropriate role of cryosurgery as a viable means of treating prostate cancer are ongoing. Cohen, Miller, Ahmed, Lotz, and Baust (2008) showed that cryosurgery alone (N = 370) resulted in a biochemical disease-free survival rate of 80.56% for low-risk patients,

74.16% for moderate-risk patients, and 45.54% for high-risk patients, indicating that cryosurgery may be as effective as other methods of treatment.

Chemotherapy

Chemotherapy for prostate cancer has historically been used for palliation following the failure of hormone manipulation in controlling the disease. Many chemotherapeutic agents have been evaluated in numerous clinical trials for the treatment of prostate cancer, including estramustine, vinblastine, vincristine, etoposide, paclitaxel, epirubicin, mitomycin C, methotrexate, cisplatin, cyclophosphamide, 5-fluorouracil, and doxorubicin. These agents have demonstrated very little clinical benefit and have not substantially improved overall survival or progression-free survival (Shelley et al., 2006). Some agents, however, have shown limited activity as single-agent therapy or as part of combination therapy. See Figure 4-4 for principles of chemotherapy as put forth by NCCN (2007).

Docetaxel

Docetaxel 75 mg/m^2 every three weeks plus prednisone 5 mg BID (arm 1) was evaluated against docetaxel 30 mg/m^2 weekly (five of six weeks) plus prednisone 5 mg BID (arm 2) and against mitoxantrone 12 mg/m^2 every three weeks plus prednisone 5 mg BID (arm 3) in a clinical trial completed by Tannock et al. (2004) (N = 1,006). Docetaxel every three weeks was found to be superior to the weekly docetaxel arm and the mitoxantrone arm, demonstrating improvement in both quality of life (13% of patients reported improvement for mitoxantrone, 22% for every-three-week docetaxel, and 23% for weekly docetaxel) and overall survival (16.5 months for mitoxantrone, 18.9 months for every-three-week docetaxel, and 17.4 months for weekly docetaxel). The weekly arm of docetaxel showed no decrease in adverse events over the every-three-week arm. Updated survival statistics from this study were reported by Berthold et al. (2008). By March 2007, data on 310 additional deaths of patients were obtained. The survival benefit of docetaxel administered every three weeks and prednisone compared with mitoxantrone administered every three weeks and prednisone had persisted with extended follow-up (p = .004). Median survival was 19.2 months in arm 1, 17.8 months in arm 2, and 16.3 months in arm 3. Trends in survival between treatment arms were seen for men greater than and less than 65 years of age, for those with and without pain at baseline, and for those with baseline PSA greater than and less than the median value of 115 ng/ml.

Estramustine

This oral antineoplastic agent has shown a 19%–69% response rate against prostate cancer when given alone. Like es-

---

Figure 4-4. National Comprehensive Cancer Network Principles of Chemotherapy

- Systemic chemotherapy should be reserved for patients with castration-recurrent metastatic prostate cancer except when studied in clinical trials.
- In this group of patients, docetaxel-based regimens have been shown to confer a survival benefit in two phase III studies:
  - SWOG 9916 compared docetaxel plus estramustine to mitoxantrone plus prednisone. Median survival for the docetaxel arm was 18 months vs. 15 months for the mitoxantrone arm (p = .01).
  - TAX 327 compared two docetaxel schedules (weekly and every 3 weeks) to mitoxantrone and prednisone. Median survival for the every 3 week docetaxel arm was 18.9 months vs. 16.5 months for the mitoxantrone arm (p = .009).
- Docetaxel-based regimens are now the standard of care for first-line treatment in this group of patients.
- Bisphosphonate therapy should be considered in patients with castration-recurrent metastatic prostate cancer since it may prevent skeletal-related events and improve bone mineral density. Bisphosphonate therapy can cause renal insufficiency and mandibular osteonecrosis in men with dental disease.
- Bisphosphonate therapy does not have a role in oncologic treatment of men with newly diagnosed, advanced prostate cancer although clinical trials are in progress.

Note. Reproduced with permission from *The NCCN 2.2007 Prostate Cancer Clinical Practice Guidelines in Oncology.* © National Comprehensive Cancer Network, 2007. Available at http://www.nccn.org. Accessed January 29, 2008. To view the most recent and complete version of the guideline, go online to www.nccn.org.

These Guidelines are a work in progress that will be refined as often as new significant data become available.

The NCCN Guidelines are a statement of consensus of its authors regarding their views of currently accepted approaches to treatment. Any clinician seeking to apply or consult any NCCN guideline is expected to use independent medical judgment in the context of individual clinical circumstances to determine any patient's care or treatment. The National Comprehensive Cancer Network makes no warranties of any kind whatsoever regarding their content, use or application and disclaims any responsibility for their application or use in any way.

---

trogens, estramustine has been linked to increased risk of DVT, pulmonary embolus, and other cardiovascular events—most of which can be prevented with prophylactic use of warfarin. Although estramustine has some benefits when used alone, it typically is used in combination with other medications. In a study completed by Eymard et al. (2007), docetaxel at 70 mg/m^2 plus estramustine at 250 mg BID days 1–5 every three weeks was compared with docetaxel at 75 mg/m^2 alone every three weeks. Of the 91 patients treated, 68% of the patients on the combination arm experienced a PSA reduction of 50% or more, compared to 30% of patients in the docetaxel-alone arm. Time to progression and median survival were longer in the combination arm than in the docetaxel-alone arm, although the study was not powered to produce statistically significant results. The Southwest Oncology Group 9916 study compared the use of mitoxantrone and prednisone to docetaxel and estramustine and found a significant improvement in overall survival in the docetaxel/estramustine group. This study did not use prophylactic warfarin, and 14.3% of patients experienced a grade 3 or 4 cardiovascular event (Eymard et al.).

Mitoxantrone

Mitoxantrone was the first chemotherapeutic agent to show improved quality of life in patients with prostate cancer. In a Canadian clinical trial comparing mitoxantrone plus prednisone versus prednisone alone, no benefit in overall survival was seen (Osoba, Tannock, Ernst, & Neville, 1999; Tannock et al., 1996). In the Tannock study ($N = 161$), 29% of patients who received mitoxantrone ($12 mg/m^2$) and prednisone experienced a palliative response, compared to 12% on prednisone alone. If the patients had worsening pain on prednisone alone after six weeks, they were crossed over to mitoxantrone plus prednisone. Fifty patients crossed over to the mitoxantrone arm, and 22% of those experienced a response. The FDA approved mitoxantrone for palliative treatment of metastatic prostate cancer pain in 1996.

Corticosteroids

Although typically used in combination with mitoxantrone, docetaxel, and ketoconazole, corticosteroids showed improved quality of life and reduced pain in 38% of patients with advanced prostate cancer when taken alone at 7.5–10 mg daily (Tannock et al., 1989). Corticosteroids also have shown significant reduction of PSA in patients with prostate cancer (Lam, Leppert, Vemulapalli, Shvarts, & Belldegrun, 2006; Storlie et al., 1995). Corticosteroids have shown limited activity in single-agent trials, which prompted them to be investigated along with other agents. Currently, corticosteroids are used mainly in combination docetaxel- and mitoxantrone-based regimens.

Future Agents

Many clinical trials are currently examining new combinations and new treatment schedules of the previously described treatment modalities. In addition, trials utilizing a number of targeted therapies are also under way. A large phase III clinical trial (Cancer and Leukemia Group B 90401) currently is comparing docetaxel with bevacizumab versus docetaxel with placebo in the treatment of HRPC (National Institutes of Health, 2007).

Satraplatin (JM216) (Spectrum Pharmaceuticals, Inc.) is a new oral platinum-based chemotherapy agent being studied in clinical trials in combination with prednisone. It was shown to have a progression-free survival of 5.2 months in combination with prednisone, compared to 2.5 months in the prednisone-alone arm in patients with HRPC with no prior chemotherapy treatments. It is dosed between 80–120 mg/m^2 daily for five days every three to five weeks. The maximum tolerated dose is 140 $mg/m^2/day$. The most common side effects include nausea and myelosuppression. Unlike cisplatin and carboplatin, it has not yet been shown to cause nephrotoxicities or neurotoxicities (McKeage, 2007).

Other recent trials have examined the efficacy of the epothilones—ixabepilone and patupilone—for the treatment of prostate cancer and HRPC. A recent review has demonstrated that these agents have potent antitumor activity in vitro and in experimental animal models of prostate cancer. In clinical studies, epothilones have no cross-resistance with taxanes and a manageable toxicity profile. Phase II studies of single-agent ixabepilone in patients with HRPC have reported a confirmed PSA response rate of 33%. In addition, higher PSA response rates have been reported in studies that assessed the use of ixabepilone with estramustine in patients with HRPC (Dawson, 2007).

Multiple trials also are looking at the effectiveness of vaccine therapy in the treatment of early-stage prostate cancer as well as HRPC.

Radiation Therapy

EBRT, the use of high-energy x-rays to kill tumor cells, is one of the standard treatment options available for clinically localized prostate cancer. In general, cancer cells are more sensitive to radiation than normal cells. When ionizing radiation is directed toward an organ, whether from external beam radiation or brachytherapy, it is absorbed by cells and permanently damages DNA in an attempt to kill malignant cells (Dewey & Bedford, 2004). The key target-molecule in the nucleus of the cell for radiation damage is believed to be DNA (Dewey & Bedford). One form of damage involves the alteration or loss of one or more of the four nitrogen-containing bases: adenine, thymine, cytosine, and guanine. A second form of damage may involve the destruction of hydrogen bonds between adenine-thymine and cytosine-guanine base pairs, which function to keep the two DNA strands together. Other damage includes breaks in one or both chains of the DNA molecule and cross-linking of the chains after breakage. When the strands are broken, resulting in damage to the DNA, consequences can vary. Major or minor effects on protein synthesis may occur, resulting in a change in the genetic material of the cell or mutation, thus resulting in impaired cellular function and cell death (Gosselin-Acomb, 2005).

Other cellular structures that are both direct and indirect targets of radiation include chromosomes, which play a key role in various stages of cellular mitosis; cell plasma and cell membrane; mitochondrial and lysosomal membranes; and cellular components such as proteins, enzymes, carbohydrates, and lipids. The combined effects of damage to chromosomes and other cellular components may contribute to the ultimate effect of radiation at the cellular level.

Historically, radiation therapy was given to the prostate by Pasteau in 1911 by inserting radium seeds through a catheter into the prostatic urethra (Pasteau & Degrais, 1913). This was shortly followed by Barringer implanting radioactive needles in 1917. It was not until years later that the first linear accelerator for treating cancer was developed by Henry Kaplan and Edward Gintzon at Stanford University in 1960. Reports flourished in the 1960s of the use of supervoltage equipment resulting in increased survival rates (Bennett, 1968; Del Regato, 1967; George, Carlton, Dykhuizen, & Dillon, 1965).

Patient Selection

EBRT should be offered to those patients with stage I, II, or III disease. Patients staged according to American Joint Committee on Cancer's staging as T1 (normal digital rectal examination [DRE]), T2 (abnormal DRE but no evidence of disease beyond confines of the prostate), and T3 (tumor extends through the prostatic capsule and possibly into the seminal vesicles) can be offered radiation therapy as definitive treatment (Greene et al., 2002; NCCN, 2007). Treatment decisions become complicated with stage T4 disease, as the tumor has invaded or is fixed to adjacent structures (i.e., bladder, external sphincter, rectum, levator muscles, or pelvic walls). Radiation therapy also may be offered to patients who are poor candidates for radical prostatectomy. See Figure 4-5 for principles of radiation therapy for prostate cancer as put forth by NCCN.

Patients who are offered radiation therapy should be further stratified by risk groups (see Table 4-3). Low-risk patients treated with either modern radiation therapy (three-dimensional conformal radiation therapy [3-D CRT], intensity-modulated radiation therapy [IMRT], or interstitial brachytherapy) or radical prostatectomy have similar progression-free survival rates (Potters et al., 2004). Standard radiation doses for low-risk patients are 70–75 Gy (NCCN, 2007). Moderate- and high-risk patients are offered EBRT with either short-term (six months) or long-term (two years) ADT. Patient selection is dependent on GS and PSA. Radiation doses for this subset of patients range from 75–80 Gy (NCCN).

Although cure certainly is possible for patients who receive EBRT, this modality has pros and cons over surgical intervention. Advantages include avoiding complications related to surgery (e.g., infection, bleeding, effects from anesthesia), low risk of urinary incontinence and stricture, better possibility of short-term preservation of erectile functioning,

Figure 4-5. National Comprehensive Cancer Network Principles of Radiation Therapy

External Beam Radiotherapy:
- 3D conformal or IMRT (intensity modulated radiation therapy) techniques should be employed.
- Doses of 70–75 Gy in 35–41 fractions to the prostate (± seminal vesicles for part of the therapy) appear to be appropriate for patients with low-risk cancers. For patients with intermediate- or high-risk disease, doses between 75–80 Gy appear to provide improved PSA-assessed disease control.
- Patients with high-risk cancers are candidates for pelvic lymph node irradiation and the addition of neoadjuvant ± adjuvant androgen ablation therapy.
- If target (PTV) margins are reduced, such as for doses above 75 Gy, extra attention to daily prostate localization, with techniques such as ultrasound, implanted fiducials, or an endorectal balloon, is indicated.

Brachytherapy:
- Permanent brachytherapy as monotherapy is indicated for patients with low-risk cancers. For intermediate-risk cancers, consider combining brachytherapy with EBRT (40–50 Gy) ± neoadjuvant androgen ablation. Patients with high-risk cancers are generally considered poor candidates for permanent brachytherapy; however, with the addition of EBRT and androgen ablation, it may be effective in select patients.
- Patients with a large prostate (> 60 g), symptoms of bladder outlet obstruction (IPSS score > 15), or a previous transurethral resection of the prostate (TURP) are not ideal candidates because of increased risk of urinary morbidity. Neoadjuvant androgen ablation may be used to shrink the prostate to an acceptable size.
- Post-implant dosimetry should be performed to document the quality of the implant.
- The recommended prescribed doses for monotherapy are 145 Gy for 125-Iodine and 125 Gy for 103-Palladium. The corresponding boost doses after 40–50 Gy EBRT are 110 Gy and 100 Gy, respectively.

Note. Reproduced with permission from *The NCCN 2.2007 Prostate Cancer Clinical Practice Guidelines in Oncology.* © National Comprehensive Cancer Network, 2007. Available at http://www.nccn.org. Accessed January 29, 2008. To view the most recent and complete version of the guideline, go online to www.nccn.org.

These Guidelines are a work in progress that will be refined as often as new significant data become available.

The NCCN Guidelines are a statement of consensus of its authors regarding their views of currently accepted approaches to treatment. Any clinician seeking to apply or consult any NCCN guideline is expected to use independent medical judgment in the context of individual clinical circumstances to determine any patient's care or treatment. The National Comprehensive Cancer Network makes no warranties of any kind whatsoever regarding their content, use or application and disclaims any responsibility for their application or use in any way.

These Guidelines are copyrighted by the National Comprehensive Cancer Network. All rights reserved. These Guidelines and illustrations herein may not be reproduced in any form for any purpose without the express written permission of the NCCN.

Table 4-3. Candidates for Radiation Therapy and Radiation Therapy With Androgen Deprivation				
Risk Category	Risk of Recurrence	Gleason Score	Prostate-Specific Antigen Level	Treatment
Low risk	80%–90% 5-year biochemical relapse-free survival	2–6	< 10 ng/ml	External beam radiation/brachytherapy
Moderate risk	50%–70% 5-year biochemical relapse-free survival	7	10–20 ng/ml	External beam radiation with short-term androgen deprivation therapy (4–6 months)
High risk	25%–33% 5-year biochemical relapse-free survival	8–10	> 20 ng/ml	External beam radiation with long-term androgen deprivation therapy (2 years)

Note. Based on information from D'Amico et al., 1999; National Comprehensive Cancer Network, 2007; Thompson et al., 2007.

and rare incidence of long-term serious side effects (Potosky et al., 2004). Disadvantages of EBRT include long length of treatment (seven to nine weeks, Monday through Friday), acute bladder or bowel symptoms, erectile dysfunction, and increased difficulty of future surgical intervention should recurrence occur (Potosky et al.). Contraindications to EBRT include history of inflammatory bowel disease (e.g., Crohn disease, ulcerative colitis); history of prior pelvic radiotherapy; or severe urinary obstructive symptoms, which may require permanent or intermittent urinary catheterization (NCCN, 2007; Thompson et al., 2007). Randomized trials directly comparing EBRT, brachytherapy, or both radiation modalities and radical prostatectomy are lacking because of the changing treatment techniques over the years and the absence of long-term clinical follow-up data that show an effect on survival rates (Jani & Hellman, 2003). However, retrospective studies with men having clinically localized disease have reported the cure rates with radiation therapy and surgery to be comparable for the first five to eight years following treatment (Kupelian et al., 2004).

Therefore, the patient and family members must understand patient selection (see Table 4-3) and the possible acute and long-term side effects of radiation therapy, whether external beam (see Figure 4-6) or brachytherapy. Whatever the method of delivery, the radiation dose needed to destroy prostate cancer cells carries the possibility of adversely affecting adjacent structures (i.e., the rectum and bladder). Only after undergoing a thorough informed consent procedure can a patient make a decision regarding choice of treatment.

Conventional External Beam Radiation Therapy

Prior to advanced planning and treatment techniques, prostate cancer was treated with radiation therapy by means that are now considered rather rudimentary. In the 1970s and 1980s, two-dimensional treatment plans were designed to treat the prostate, continuing to kill cells with high-energy x-rays. Lead blocks shielded the surrounding healthy tissues. Patients were treated with a four-field technique: anterior/posterior and posterior/anterior directions. This technique gradually evolved to include six fields with the addition of right and left lateral oblique fields. Despite good intentions, these methods resulted in severe toxicities and a high degree of morbidity. The radiation dose generally was around 60 Gy (Perez, Bauer, Garza, & Royce, 1977). Treatment utilizing this technique allowed physicians the limited ability to localize the prostate, as soft-tissue structures were not well visualized.

However, when advances in computed tomography (CT) and nuclear medicine occurred in the 1980s and 1990s, the delivery of therapeutic radiation dramatically changed. Developing around the same time was the improved ability to deliver and focus beams of radiation produced by newer-generation linear accelerators. CT greatly improve the ability to visualize anatomic structures, including the prostate. When CT images are merged with updated treatment planning and treatment administration software, the accuracy of radiation therapy is greatly improved. Changes from the two-dimensional treatment plan to 3-D CRT enhanced the ability to identify the prostate and pelvic structures. Conformal radiation therapy allows shaping of the radiation beam to match the corresponding shape of the target, thus reducing the amount of radiation received by healthy surrounding tissues. As a result, side effect profiles are decreased, allowing delivery of higher doses of radiation and ultimately affecting survival rates (Herman et al., 2003).

Three-Dimensional Conformal Radiation Therapy

3-D CRT evolved from conventional (two-dimensional) external beam radiation as newer computer software was developed. Merging newer imaging technology with radiation oncology software and equipment has allowed more precise 3-D CRT and more clearly defined treatment fields. Radiation oncologists are now able to outline prostate, seminal vesicles, bladder, rectum, and femoral heads during the planning phase of treatment. Computer software then generates a 3-D repre-

Figure 4-6. Major Physiologic Side Effects of External Beam Radiation Therapy				
Urinary	**Bowel**	**Sexual Dysfunction**	**Fatigue**	**Myelosuppression**
Acute • Dysuria • Frequency • Hesitancy • Urgency • Hematuria • Vascular changes to bladder • Reduced bladder capacity **Acute and Chronic/ Long-Term** • Hematuria (caused by mucosal inflammation) • Cystitis	**Acute** • Diarrhea • Tenesmus • Proctalgia • Bleeding • Abdominal cramps **Acute and Chronic/ Long-Term** • Diarrhea • Fistulas • Perforation • Obstruction • Bleeding • Fibrosis	**Acute and Chronic/ Long-Term** • Erectile dysfunction • Impotence	**Acute and Chronic/ Long-Term** • Temporary • Multifactorial	**Acute and Chronic/ Long-Term** • Seen with large pelvic fields • Radiation combined with chemotherapy

Potential exists for acute side effects to last into the chronic phase (> 30 days post-treatment).

Note. Based on information from Hogle, 2007.

sentation of all these structures and their spatial relationship to one another. The radiation oncologist and physics team then use this information to customize beams that more accurately target the area of disease while minimizing exposure to normal tissue. This greatly increased confidence in the target area and resulted in smaller treatment fields, which eventually led to dosage ranges between 70–78 Gy (Hanks, Hanlon, Epstein, & Horwitz, 2002; Khoo, 2005). The current radiation dosage range recommended by NCCN (2007) is 70–80 Gy.

Significant strides in radiation dose escalation have demonstrated survival benefits. Zietman et al. (2005) conducted a randomized controlled trial of 393 patients at Loma Linda University Medical Center and Massachusetts General Hospital. Patients with early-stage prostate cancer (T1b through T2b) with a PSA level less than 15 ng/ml were randomized to a total dose of either 70.2 Gy (conventional dose) or 79.2 Gy (high dose). A combination of conformal photon and proton beams was utilized. The results revealed that men with clinically localized prostate cancer had a lower risk of biochemical failure if treated with a higher dose of radiation (79.2 Gy). This study supported an earlier phase III randomized trial from M.D. Anderson by Pollack et al. (2002) that compared doses of 70 Gy to doses of 78 Gy. These investigators found that increasing the total dose by 8 Gy resulted in a significant improvement in the failure rates for patients with intermediate-to-high risk of disease. Studies also have shown that 3-D CRT has offered superior control of the radiation dose, thus enabling radiation oncologists to deliver higher doses safely as well (Zapatero, Rios, Marin, Minguez, & Garcia-Vecente, 2006).

The development of the multileaf collimator significantly influenced the improvement of 3-D CRT. Upon their refine-

ment and implementation during the 1990s, multileaf collimators changed the process of delivering radiation therapy. Previously, heavy custom-made lead blocks were cut and molded for each treatment field. The blocks were hoisted and fixed into place on a linear accelerator to block or shape portions of the radiation beam. Now, a multileaf collimator, which consists of a series of independent metal "leaves" made of a tungsten alloy, are manufactured and installed directly into the linear accelerator. The leaves are arranged via computer programming according to the patient's treatment plan and by physician discretion. The multileaf collimator essentially has the same effect as a custom lead or cerrobend block but avoids the tedious process and physical strain of custom-making and positioning each block (see Figure 4-7). Multileaf collimators currently are used with 3-D CRT and IMRT as well.

Intensity-Modulated Radiation Therapy

In the 21st century, an even newer therapeutic radiation technique, IMRT, is available. IMRT allows for the variation of radiation dose to a target, in this case the prostate, and the surrounding tissue, thus further decreasing toxicity to the bladder, small bowel, and rectum while allowing for dose escalation. The intensity of the beam is modulated intentionally, allowing for therapeutic radiation doses of 70–80 Gy (NCCN, 2007). IMRT is a further evolution of 3-D CRT. The two main goals of IMRT are to spare normal tissue by reducing toxicity to surrounding areas and to improve cancer control and cure by delivering intensified and often escalated doses of radiation to the designated target. IMRT is unique in that it can deliver radiation from multiple beam angles while allowing for varia-

Figure 4-7. Multileaf Collimator

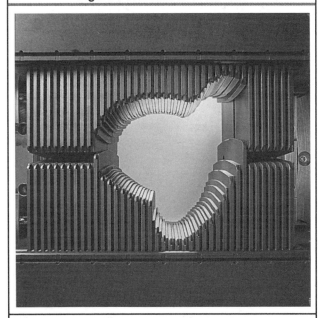

The multileaf collimator can be programmed to shape the beam of radiation to conform to most tumors.

Note. Photo courtesy of Varian Medical Systems of Palo Alto, CA. All rights reserved.

tion in the intensity of the radiation beam across the target area. In comparison to other delivery systems (conventional or 3-D CRT), IMRT has demonstrated an 80% decrease in overall toxicity to patients being treated for prostate cancer and an increase in disease-free survival (Zelefsky, Valicenti, Goodman, & Perez, 2002). IMRT's dosimetry offers increased dose heterogeneity to target and normal tissues and allows for a reduction in treatment margins relative to 3-D CRT and conventional radiation, thus increasing tumor control probability (Luxton, Hancock, & Boyer, 2004).

With the advent of IMRT allowing for dose escalation, image-guidance radiotherapy provides an important advantage when having to account for organ movement. Currently, multiple technologies exist to allow accurate localization of the prostate gland just prior to treatment. These technologies include transabdominal ultrasound, endorectal balloon ultrasound, or placement of interstitial fiducial markers into the gland itself. The gold fiducial markers are easily visualized via fluoroscopy, which is available on certain linear accelerators. Placement of the interstitial markers is a relatively minor invasive procedure done either in the operating room or the physician's office. Specially trained radiation therapists can isolate the prostate gland by using the previously described ultrasound techniques. All of these prostate localization methods are used in conjunction with the precise CT-guided treatment planning techniques and with 3-D CRT or IMRT. They are an additional measure of target confirmation and allow for

last-minute treatment adjustments just prior to "beam on" to account for any organ movement. These described target confirmation techniques have the potential to improve local control and reduce late radiation-related sequelae.

TomoTherapy

The next generation of cutting-edge technology in radiation therapy is the TomoTherapy® (TomoTherapy Inc.) system. Unlike earlier methods of utilizing relatively large beams of radiation from multiple different directions, TomoTherapy uses hundreds of pencil-thin beams of radiation from multiple directions while spirally rotating around the tumor. The patient moves through treatment in a unit similar to a CT scanner, but instead of regular x-rays, a series of special high-energy x-rays are spirally rotated around the patient. The intent is to deliver high doses to the tumor while reducing the dose to normal organs with a goal of significantly reducing side effects. Clinical trials currently are under way to compare helical TomoTherapy utilizing IMRT versus conventional 3-D CRT (Ramsey et al., 2007).

Proton Beam Therapy

Proton beam therapy is a type of conformal therapy that bombards the target area with protons instead of x-rays. Proton irradiation has proved effective in the treatment of benign and malignant disease (Verhey & Munzenrider, 1982). A proton is a positively charged particle in the nucleus of all atoms, which relates to that atom's atomic number. In order to generate and administer proton beam therapy, a cyclotron must be used. A cyclotron is essentially a nuclear reactor capable of smashing atoms to release charged ions, some of which are protons. The use of proton beam therapy is not widely available. Excessive space requirements and cost of installation have limited the number of proton beam centers worldwide. The value of using protons as a clinical tool include allowance for greater precision and control; minimal amount of scatter radiation; characteristic distribution of treatment dose and depth; and most of the energy from protons is deposited near the end of their target range (Leaver & Alfred, 2004). Vargas et al. (2008) at the University of Florida Proton Therapy Institute evaluated patients with low-risk disease. Patients were treated with 78 Gy, and when compared to IMRT, proton therapy reduced the dose to adjacent structures while maintaining target coverage volume. Long-term results need time to decipher freedom from failure. Trofimov et al. (2007) also were able to design lower treatment prescriptions with proton therapy, but again, final long-range outcomes are yet to be determined.

Interstitial Brachytherapy

Over the past century, brachytherapy has evolved to become a widely used modality for the treatment of early-stage prostate cancer. Interstitial prostate brachytherapy involves placing radioactive sources into the prostatic tissue through needles, seeds, or wires via transrectal ultrasound guidance. Brachytherapy may be used as the sole form of radiation therapy, or it may be used in combination with EBRT. Gaining in popularity, brachytherapy for early, clinically organ-confined prostate cancer can be administered as monotherapy with excellent outcomes (Thompson et al., 2007). This would include patients with T1c–T2a, GS 2–6, and a PSA level less than 10 ng/ml. See Figure 4-8 for additional criteria when considering brachytherapy as primary treatment for a patient with prostate cancer. Two delivery techniques exist for prostate brachytherapy: low-dose-rate (LDR) and high-dose-rate (HDR).

Figure 4-8. Candidates for Interstitial Brachytherapy

- T1 or T2a disease
- Low Gleason score (GS) (2–6)
- Low prostate-specific antigen (PSA) level (< 10 ng/ml)
- Prostate size 20–60 g
- No bladder outlet obstruction (international prostate symptom score > 15)
- No history of transurethral resection of the prostate or, if distant history, minimal defect in the gland as confirmed by transrectal ultrasound
- Consideration as a boost with external beam radiation (T2b–T2c, GS of 7, or PSA level of 10–20 ng/ml)

Note. Based on information from National Comprehensive Cancer Network, 2007; Thompson et al., 2007.

Low-Dose-Rate Brachytherapy

The radioactive sources most frequently utilized in permanent prostate brachytherapy, also known as LDR, are iodine-125 (^{125}I) and palladium-103 (^{103}Pd). More recently, some centers are using cesium (^{131}Cs). Although no clinical data exist that demonstrate an advantage of one permanent source over another, differences in half-life and dose rate suggest that ^{125}I is better suited for slow-growing, low-grade tumors, whereas ^{103}Pd may be better suited for high-grade disease. The half-life of ^{125}I is 60 days, ^{103}Pd has a half-life of 17 days, and ^{131}Cs has a half-life of just less than 10 days. ^{131}Cs also has a higher dose rate than ^{125}I or ^{103}Pd, allowing for the delivery of more radiation over a shorter period of time. Because the use of ^{131}Cs in this patient population is relatively new, outcome data are limited. Long-term data examining biochemical relapse-free survival rates traditionally have been focused on patients who received ^{125}I or ^{103}Pd implants. Of these patients, LDR brachytherapy as primary treatment has yielded 85%–94% relapse-free survival rates for low-risk disease, 77%–84% for intermediate-risk disease, and 45%–54% for high-risk disease (Blasko, Grimm, Sylvester, & Cavanagh, 2000; Grimm, Blasko, Sylvester, Meier, & Cavanagh, 2001;

Kollmeier, Stock, & Stone, 2003; Murphy et al., 2004; Sylvester, Blasko, Grimm, Meier, & Malmgren, 2003).

The actual technique involves placement of the radioactive source into the prostate gland during an operative procedure while the patient is under general or spinal anesthesia. Once anesthetized, the patient is placed in a dorsal lithotomy position and a grid or template is positioned against the perineum. A transrectal ultrasound probe then is inserted into the rectum. Ultrasound images allow for visualization of the prostate while needles are placed directly into the gland. The needles are either preloaded with radioactive seeds or attached to a Mick® (C.R. Bard, Inc.) applicator that deposits the radioactive seeds into the gland. Dosimetry planning, done at the time of implant or days to weeks prior, is used to determine the exact placement of the seeds. Typically, seeds are distributed throughout the prostate, approximately 1 cm apart. Generally, 80–100 seeds are deposited into the prostate gland, although the exact number depends on the strength of the seeds and the size of the gland. The usual prescribed dose for implant alone with ^{125}I is 145 Gy, and ^{103}Pd is 125 Gy (NCCN, 2007; Zelefsky et al., 2004).

In patients with higher-grade prostate tumors, brachytherapy alone is considered insufficient treatment, as this typically results in underdosing the prostate and surrounding tissues. Higher-grade tumors require a higher total dose of radiation. Combining brachytherapy with EBRT offers an effective approach for patients with high-grade disease. When receiving combined treatment, the patient generally receives 45–50 Gy of EBRT to the prostate gland in conjunction with a low-dose boost of 90 Gy if using ^{103}Pd and 110 Gy if using ^{125}I. Clinical evidence supporting the use of EBRT before or after seed implant is lacking. Further, no evidence exists to support the use of ^{125}I over ^{103}Pd when considering combined treatment. Finally, EBRT following permanent seed implant has not been shown to significantly increase overall morbidity versus EBRT alone (Kestin et al., 2000; Zelefsky et al., 2004).

High-Dose-Rate Brachytherapy

HDR prostate brachytherapy typically utilizes an iridium source (^{192}Ir) to deliver a therapeutic dose of radiation. HDR, like LDR, also can be administered as primary treatment alone or in combination with EBRT. Similar to permanent seed implantation (LDR), ultrasound-guided imagery is used to guide the placement of needles into the prostate gland while the patient is under the effects of anesthesia (general or spinal). Either the needles or plastic catheters are left behind to act as a vessel for the iridium source. Different from LDR, in which seeds are permanently placed, HDR treatment is delivered by placing the source directly into the prostate gland via these needles or plastic catheters and then removed. After CT-based treatment planning, several high-dose fractions (treatments) ranging from 4–6 Gy are administered over an interval of 24–36 hours. Depending on the strength of the iridium source, each fraction can last 5–15 minutes, after which the source is removed. This modality may be followed by EBRT to a dose of 45–50 Gy. Some clinicians have performed prostate HDR treatments throughout the course of EBRT and have examined the efficacy of dose escalation per fraction of HDR treatments. Improved outcomes were observed compared with the outcomes of using lower dose levels (Kestin et al., 2000; Martinez, 2000).

Once the patient agrees to undergo brachytherapy, the decision to utilize HDR or LDR ultimately rests with the physician. Training and personal preference are factors that often determine physician choice of one type of brachytherapy source over another. Side effect profiles for LDR and HDR brachytherapy are similar (see Figure 4-9). Some argue that an HDR after-loading approach allows for limiting under-dosed areas within the gland. Zelefsky et al. (2004) reported that HDR offers a higher rate of tumor cell kill, which can be advantageous in patients with bulky tumors or adverse prognostic features.

Figure 4-9. Side Effects* of Interstitial Brachytherapy

Urinary
- Dysuria
- Frequency
- Urgency
- Difficulty starting or interrupted stream
- Retention
- Hematuria
- Increased nocturia

Bowel
- Diarrhea

Scrotal/Perineal Discomfort
- Caused by bleeding ecchymoses

Sexual Dysfunction
- Erectile dysfunction
- Semen discoloration

Proctitis
- Small, gassy bowel movements
- Painless rectal bleeding
- Rectal irritation

*These generally are viewed as temporary side effects that may last several months after implantation, with the exception of erectile dysfunction, which can be a long-term effect.

Note. Based on information from Hogle, 2007; Thompson et al., 2007.

Radiopharmaceuticals

Another type of radiation therapy is referred to as radio-pharmaceutical or radionuclide therapy (RPT). This type of treatment utilizes unsealed radioactive sources in a liquid or colloidal suspension to treat specific tumors. In treating patients with prostate cancer, RPT is reserved for the palliative

treatment of metastatic bone disease, which often is the result of advanced prostate cancer. In 1941, Charles Pecher, a then graduate student at the University of California, Berkeley, was the first to demonstrate uptake of radiopharmaceuticals (strontium-89 [^{89}Sr] and phosphorus-32) in bone by means of x-rays. Later in 1942, he injected ^{89}Sr to systemically treat patients with skeletal metastatic disease from prostate cancer with excellent clinical response. Unfortunately, he died later that same year in World War II. After his death, his work went silent until regaining recognition in 1974. Finally, in 1993, ^{89}Sr received FDA approval. In 1997, a second radiopharmaceutical received approval for palliation of bone pain arising from bone metastases, samarium-153 (^{153}Sm). Resche et al. (1997) conducted a randomized, dose-controlled study of efficacy and safety of samarium. Of the 114 patients studied, 67 had prostate cancer. Although statistics were not subdivided per cancer site, improvement occurred in the degree of pain, level of daytime discomfort, quality of sleep, and pain relief.

Today, men with locally advanced prostate cancer (i.e., bone metastases) can benefit from RPT (see Figure 4-10). Different from EBRT, this approach injects a radioactive substance, ^{89}Sr or ^{153}Sm, directly into the vein (Maini, Sciuto, Romano, & Bergomi, 2003). These substances have an affinity for areas of the bone that contain malignant cancer cells through various mechanisms. ^{89}Sr isolates calcium deposits that typically occur following osteoclastic lesions. ^{153}Sm, once injected, chemically adds a phosphoric acid group and is drawn to sites where newly deposited bone tissue has formed (Maini et al.).

Figure 4-10. Candidates for Radiopharmaceuticals

Strontium-89 (Metastron™, GE Healthcare)
- Patient has widely disseminated prostate cancer not amenable to localized therapy.
- Primary management with hormonal manipulation has failed.
- Strontium-89 is contraindicated in patients with renal insufficiency (abnormal blood urea nitrogen [BUN]/creatinine).
- Platelet count is ideally around 100,000 but can be as low as 60,000.
- White blood cell count is ideally 4,000 but can be as low as 2,400.

Samarium-153 (Quadramet®, Cytogen Corp.)
- Patient has widely disseminated prostate cancer and osteoblastic metastatic bone lesions confirmed by x-ray films and radionuclide bone scan.
- Patient has no known hypersensitivity to EDTMP compound or similar phosphonate compounds.
- Samarium-153 is contraindicated in patients with renal insufficiency (abnormal BUN/creatinine).
- White blood cell counts and platelet counts can decrease to a nadir of approximately 40%–50% of baseline within 3–5 weeks after administration and tend to return to pretreatment levels by 8 weeks.

Note. Based on information from Baczyk et al., 2007; DrugLib.com, 2006.

The main differences between ^{89}Sr and [153]Sm are the half-life of each isotope (50.5 days and 1.9 days, respectively), beta-ray energy emissions (0.58 and 0.22 MeV, respectively), and depth of penetration (2.4 mm and 0.55 mm, respectively). These differences influence the potential side effects that one might experience, which include thrombocytopenia, decreased white blood cell count, and transient bone pain associated with a "flare" reaction after administration (Kossman & Weiss, 2000; Temple, 2007). Pain relief with ^{89}Sr typically is seen in 7–20 days. During their investigation, Baczyk et al. (2007) studied 60 male patients treated with ^{89}Sr versus [153]Sm. Although both provided relief, the pain relief was better for osteoblastic metastases than in patients with mixed metastases.

Conclusion

Numerous factors are considered when discussing treatment recommendations for patients with prostate cancer. In addition to staging, laboratory and diagnostic studies, factors such as patient comorbidities, personal preference, and potential side effect profiles, as well as survival rate and life expectancy, all need to be considered when making a treatment decision. The final decision regarding active surveillance, radical prostatectomy, hormonal manipulation, EBRT, or interstitial brachytherapy can be overwhelming. Such a decision can be further complicated by having to choose between surgical techniques, hormonal schedules, and type of brachytherapy (^{125}I or [103]Pd). Therefore, patients with prostate cancer must be properly educated about the treatment options available, as well as the implications associated with each option. Patients need to make informed treatment decisions in conjunction with family members and their physicians.

Studies examining new administration schedules of existing treatments and newer modalities are ongoing. As with management of many malignancies, management of prostate cancer has become similar to that of a chronic disease. When one modality fails the patient, another is used. It is hoped that the future will bring improved methods of screening and diagnosis, newer surgical techniques, and technologic advances, as well as improved cure rates for patients with prostate cancer.

References

Baczyk, M., Czepczynski, R., Milecki, P., Pisarek, M., Oleksa, R., & Sowinski, J. (2007). 89Sr versus 153Sm-EDTMP: Comparison of treatment efficacy of painful bone metastases in prostate and breast carcinoma. *Nuclear Medicine Communications, 28*(4), 245–250.

Bennett, J.E. (1968). Treatment of carcinoma of the prostate by cobalt beam therapy. *Radiology, 90*(3), 532–535.

Berry, D.L. (2004). Bladder disturbances. In C.H. Yarbro, M.H. Frogge, & M. Goodman (Eds.), *Cancer symptom management* (3rd ed., pp. 493–504). Sudbury, MA: Jones and Bartlett.

Berthold, D.R., Pond, G.R., Soban, F., de Wit, R., Eisenberger, M., & Tannock, I.F. (2008). Docetaxel plus prednisone or mitoxantrone plus prednisone for advanced prostate cancer: Updated survival in the TAX 327 study. *Journal of Clinical Oncology, 26*(2), 242–245.

Blasko, J.C., Grimm P.D., Sylvester, J.E., & Cavanagh, W. (2000). The role of external beam radiotherapy with 1-125/Pd-103 brachytherapy for prostate carcinoma. *Radiotherapy and Oncology, 57*(3), 273–278.

Bolla, M., Descotes, J., Artignan, X., & Fourneret, P. (2007). Adjuvant treatment to radiation: Combined hormone therapy and external radiotherapy for locally advanced prostate cancer. *BJU International, 100*(Suppl. 2), 44–47.

Bollens, R., Roumeguere, T., Vanden Bossche, M., Quackels, T., Zlotta, A.R., & Schulman, C.C. (2002). Comparison of laparoscopic radical prostatectomy techniques. *Current Urology Reports, 3*(2), 148–151.

Borden, L.S., & Kozlowski, P.M. (2006). Robotic assisted laparoscopic radical prostatectomy: An objective assessment and review of the literature. *Scientific World Journal, 7*(6), 2589–3061.

Bremner, K.E., Chong, C.A., Tomlinson, G., Alibhai, S.M., & Krahn, M.D. (2007). A review of meta-analysis and prostate cancer utilities. *Medical Decision Making, 27*(3), 288–298.

Bruchovsky, N., Klotz, L., Crook, J., & Goldenberg, S.L. (2007). Locally advanced prostate cancer—biochemical results from a prospective phase II study of intermittent androgen suppression for men with evidence of prostate-specific antigen recurrence after radiotherapy. *Cancer, 109*(5), 858–867.

Cathelineau, X., Arroyo, C., Rozet, F., Baumert, H., & Vallancien, G. (2004). Laparoscopic and radical prostatectomy: The new gold standard? *Current Urology Reports, 5*(2), 108–114.

Chon, J.K., Jacobs, S.C., & Naslund, M.J. (2000). The cost value of medical versus surgical hormonal therapy for metastatic prostate cancer. *Journal of Urology, 164*(3), 735–737.

Choo, R., Klotz, L., Danjoux, C., Morton, G.C., DeBoer, G., Szumacher, E., et al. (2002). Feasibility study: Watchful waiting for localized low to intermediate grade prostate carcinoma with selective delayed intervention based on prostate specific antigen, histological and/or clinical progression. *Journal of Urology, 167*(4), 1664–1669.

Clinical Pharmacology [Database online]. (2008). Tampa, FL: Gold Standard, Inc. Retrieved January 30, 2008, from http://www.clinicalpharmacology.com

Cohen, J.K., Miller, R.J., Jr., Ahmed, S., Lotz, M.J., & Baust, J. (2008). Ten-year biochemical disease control for patients with prostate cancer treated with cryosurgery as primary therapy. *Urology, 71*(3), 515–518.

D'Amico, A.V., Whittington, R., Malkowicz, S.B., Fondurulia, J., Chen, M.H., Kaplan, I., et al. (1999). Pretreatment nomogram for prostate-specific antigen recurrence after radical prostatectomy or external-beam radiation therapy for clinically localized prostate cancer. *Journal of Clinical Oncology, 17*(1), 168–172.

Dawson, N.A. (2007). Epothilones in prostate cancer: Review of clinical experience. *Annals of Oncology, 18*(Suppl. 5), 22–27.

De La Taille, A., Benson, M.C., Bagiella, E., Burchardt, M., Shabsigh, A., Olsson, C.A., et al. (2000). Cryoablation for clinically localized prostate cancer using an argon-based system: Complication rates and biochemical recurrence. *BJU International, 85*(3), 281–286.

Del Regato, J.A. (1967). Radiotherapy in the conservative treatment of operable and locally inoperable carcinoma of the prostate. *Radiology, 88*(4), 761–766.

Dewey, W.C., & Bedford, J.S. (2004). Radiobiologic principles. In S.A. Leibel & T.L. Phillips (Eds.), *Textbook of radiation oncology* (2nd ed., pp. 3–30). Philadelphia: Saunders.

Dhar, N.B., Burkhard, F.C., & Studer, V.E. (2007). Role of lymphadenectomy in clinically organ-confined prostate cancer. *World Journal of Urology, 25*(1), 39–44.

DrugLib.com. (2006, June 1). *Quadramet (samarium SM 153 lexidronam pentasodium): Warnings and precautions.* Retrieved February 1, 2008, from http://www.druglib.com/druginfo/quadramet/precautions

Eymard, J.C., Priou, F., Zannetti, A., Ravaud, A., Lepille, D., & Kerbrat, P. (2007). Randomized phase II study of docetaxel plus estramustine and single-agent docetaxel in patients with metastatic hormone-refractory prostate cancer. *Annals of Oncology, 18*(6), 1064–1070.

Frydenberg, M., & Oesterling, J.E. (1997). Management of stage C (T3) prostate cancer: Nonradiation therapy. In D. Raghavan, H.I. Scher, S.A. Leibel, & P.H. Lange (Eds.), *Principles and practice of genitourinary oncology* (pp. 535–541). Philadelphia: Lippincott-Raven.

George, F.W., Carlton, C.E., Jr., Dykhuizen, R.F., & Dillon, J.R. (1965). Cobalt-60 telecurietherapy in the definitive treatment of carcinoma of the prostate: A preliminary report. *Journal of Urology, 93,* 102–109.

Gosselin-Acomb, T.K. (2005). Principles of radiation therapy. In C.H. Yarbro, M.H. Frogge, & M. Goodman (Eds.), *Cancer nursing: Principles and practice* (6th ed., pp. 229–249). Sudbury, MA: Jones and Bartlett.

Greene, F.L., Page, D.L., Fleming, I.D., Fritz, A., Balch, C.M., Haller, D.G., et al. (Eds.). (2002). *AJCC cancer staging handbook* (6th ed.). New York: Springer.

Greenspan, S.L., Nelson, J.B., Trump, D.L., & Resnick, N.M. (2007). Effect of once-weekly oral alendronate on bone loss in men receiving androgen deprivation therapy for prostate cancer. *Annals of Internal Medicine, 146*(6), 416–424.

Grimm, P.D., Blasko, J.C., Sylvester, J.E., Meier, R.M., & Cavanagh, W. (2001). 10-year biochemical (prostate-specific antigen) control of prostate cancer with 125-I brachytherapy. *International Journal of Radiation Oncology, Biology, Physics, 51*(1), 31–40.

Hanks, G.E., Hanlon, A.L., Epstein, B., & Horwitz, E.M. (2002). Dose response in prostate cancer with 8–12 years' follow-up. *International Journal of Radiation Oncology, Biology, Physics, 54*(2), 427–435.

Held-Warmkessel, J. (2005). Prostate cancer. In C.H Yarbro, M.H. Frogge, & M. Goodman (Eds.), *Cancer nursing: Principles and practice* (6th ed., pp. 1552–1580). Sudbury, MA: Jones and Bartlett.

Herman, M.G., Pisansky, T.M., Kruse, J.J., Prisciandaro, J.I., Davis, B.J., & King, B.F. (2003). Technical aspects of daily online positioning of the prostate for three-dimensional conformal radiotherapy using an electronic portal imaging device. *International Journal of Radiation Oncology, Biology, Physics, 57*(4), 1131–1140.

Herrmann, T.R., Rabenalt, R., Stolzenburg, J.U., Liatsikos, E.N., Imkamp, F., Tezval, H., et al. (2007). Oncological and functional results of open, robot-assisted and laparoscopic radical prostatectomy: Does surgical approach and surgical experience matter? *World Journal of Urology, 25*(2), 149–160.

Hogle, W.P. (2007). Male genitourinary cancers. In M.L. Haas, W.P. Hogle, G.J. Moore-Higgs, & T.K. Gosselin-Acomb (Eds.), *Radiation therapy: A guide to patient care* (pp. 234–266). Philadelphia: Mosby.

Isaacs, J.T., Lundmo, P.I., Berges, R., Martikainen, P., Kyprianou, N., & English, H.F. (1992). Androgen regulation of programmed cell death of normal and malignant prostatic cells. *Journal of Andrology, 13*(6), 457–464.

Jani, A.B., & Hellman, S. (2003). Early prostate cancer: Clinical decision-making. *Lancet, 361*(9362), 1045–1053.

Jemal, A., Siegel, R., Ward, E., Hao, Y., Xu, J., Murray, T., et al. (2008). Cancer statistics. *CA: A Cancer Journal for Clinicians, 58*(2), 71–96.

Kestin, L.L., Martinez, A.A., Stromberg, J.S., Edmundson, G.K., Gustafson, G.S., Brabbins, D.S., et al. (2000). Matched-pair analysis of conformal high-dose rate brachytherapy boost versus external beam radiation therapy alone for locally advanced prostate cancer. *Journal of Clinical Oncology, 18*(15), 2869–2880.

Khoo, V.S. (2005). Radiotherapeutic techniques for prostate cancer, dose escalation and brachytherapy. *Clinical Oncology, 17*(7), 560–571.

Khosla, S., Burr, D., Cauley, J., Demster, D.W., Ebeling, P.R., Felsenberg, D., et al. (2007). Bisphosphonate-associated osteonecrosis of the jaw: Report of a task force of the American Society for Bone and Mineral Research. *Journal of Bone and Mineral Research, 22*(10), 1479–1492.

Kirby, R.S., Christmas, T.J., & Brawer, M.K. (2001). *Prostate cancer* (2nd ed.). London: Mosby.

Klotz, L. (2005). Active surveillance for prostate cancer: For whom? *Clinical Journal of Oncology, 23*(32), 8165–8169.

Klotz, L. (2006). Active surveillance versus radical treatment for favorable-risk localized prostate cancer. *Current Treatment Options in Oncology, 7*(5), 355–362.

Kollmeier, M.A., Stock, R.G., & Stone, N. (2003). Biochemical outcomes after prostate brachytherapy with 5-year minimal follow-up: Importance of patient selection and implant quality. *International Journal of Radiation Oncology, Biology, Physics, 57*(3), 645–653.

Kossman, S.E., & Weiss, M.A. (2000). Acute myelogenous leukemia after exposure to strontium-89 for the treatment of adenocarcinoma of the prostate cancer. *Cancer, 88*(3), 620–624.

Kupelian, P.A., Potters, L., Khuntia, D., Ciezki, J.P., Reddy, C.A., Reuther, A.M., et al. (2004). Radical prostatectomy, external beam radiotherapy < 72 Gy, external beam radiotherapy ≥ 72 Gy, permanent seed implantation, or combined seeds/external beam radiotherapy for stage T1-T2 prostate cancer. *International Journal of Radiation Oncology, Biology, Physics, 58*(1), 25–33.

Lam, J.S., Leppert, J.T., Vemulapalli, S.N., Shvarts, O., & Belldegrun, A.S. (2006). Secondary hormonal therapy for prostate cancer. *Journal of Urology, 175*(1), 27–34.

Lanfranco, A., Castellanos, A., Desai, J., & Meyers, W.C. (2004). Robotic surgery: A current perspective. *Annals of Surgery, 239*(1), 14–21.

Leaver, D., & Alfred, L. (2004). Treatment delivery equipment. In C.M. Washington & D. Leaver (Eds.), *Principles and practice of radiation therapy* (2nd ed., pp. 131–170). St. Louis, MO: Mosby.

Luxton, G., Hancock, S.L., & Boyer, A.L. (2004). Dosimetry and radiobiologic model comparison of IMRT and 3D conformal radiotherapy in treatment of carcinoma of the prostate. *International Journal of Radiation Oncology, Biology, Physics, 59*(1), 267–284.

Maini, C.L., Sciuto, R., Romano, L., & Bergomi, S. (2003). Radionuclide therapy with bone seeking radionuclides in palliation of painful bone metastases. *Journal of Experimental and Clinical Cancer Research, 22*(Suppl. 4), 71–74.

Martikainen, P., Kyprianou, N., Tucker, R.W., & Isaacs, J.T. (1991). Programmed death of nonproliferating androgen-independent prostatic cancer cells. *Cancer Research, 51*(17), 4693–4700.

Martinez, A.A. (2000). High dose rate brachytherapy for prostate cancer. In C. Greco & M.J. Zelefsky (Eds.), *Radiotherapy for prostate cancer* (pp. 279–286). Amsterdam: Harwood Academic Publishers.

Mason, T.M. (2006). Surgery. In J. Held-Warmkessel (Ed.), *Contemporary issues in prostate cancer: A nursing perspective* (2nd ed., pp. 166–182). Sudbury, MA: Jones and Bartlett.

McKeage, M.J. (2007). Satraplatin in hormone-refractory prostate cancer and other tumour types. *Drugs, 67*(6), 859–869.

McLeod, D.G. (2003). Hormonal therapy: Historical perspective to future directions. *Urology, 61*(Suppl. 2), 3–7.

McLeod, D.G., Iversen, P., See, W.A., Morris, T., Armstrong, J., & Wirth, M.P. (2006). Bicalutamide 150 mg plus standard care vs standard care alone for early prostate cancer. *BJU International, 97*(2), 247–254.

McLeod, D.G., See, W.A., Klimberg, I., Gleason, D., Chodak, G., Montie, J., et al. (2006). The bicalutamide 150 mg early prostate cancer program: Findings of the North American trial at 7.7-year median followup. *Journal of Urology, 176*(1), 75–80.

Messing, E.M., Manola, J., Yao, J., Crawford, D., Wilding, G., & Trump, D. (2006). Immediate versus deferred androgen deprivation treatment in patients with node-positive prostate cancer after radical prostatectomy and pelvic lymphadenectomy. *Lancet Oncology, 7*(6), 472–479.

Moul, J.W. (2000). Prostate specific antigen only progression of prostate cancer. *Journal of Urology, 163*(6), 1632–1642.

Murphy, M.Y., Piper, R.K., Greenwood, L.R., Mitch, M.G., Lamperti, P.J., Seltzer, S.M., et al. (2004). Evaluation of the new cesium-131 for use in low-energy x-ray brachytherapy. *Medical Physics, 31*(6), 1529–1538.

Nakabayashi, M., Xie, W., Regan, M., Jackman, D., Kantoff, P., & Oh, W. (2006). Response to low-dose ketoconazole and subsequent dose escalation to high-dose ketoconazole in patients with androgen-independent prostate cancer. *Cancer, 107*(5), 975–981.

National Comprehensive Cancer Network. (2007). *NCCN Clinical Practice Guidelines in Oncology™: Prostate cancer early detection* [v.2.2007]. Retrieved March 7, 2008, from http://www.nccn.org/professionals/physician_gls/PDF/prostate_detection.pdf

National Institutes of Health. (2007). *Prostate cancer clinical trials.* Retrieved September 30, 2007, from http://www.clinicaltrials.gov/ct/search;jsessionid=52365CE57806B259DA9F397F4DD7C1D9?term=prostate+cancer

Osoba, D., Tannock, I.F., Ernst, D.S., & Neville, A.J. (1999). Health-related quality of life in men with metastatic prostate cancer treated with prednisone alone or mitoxantrone and prednisone. *Journal of Clinical Oncology, 17*(6), 1654–1663.

Pasteau, O., & Degrais, J. (1913). De l'emploi du radium dan le traitement des cancers de la prostate. *Journal of Urology (Paris), 4,* 341–366.

Perez, C.A., Bauer, W., Garza, R., & Royce, R.K. (1977). Radiation therapy in the definitive treatment of localized carcinoma of the prostate. *Cancer, 40*(4), 1425–1433.

Pirtsvholaishvili, G., Hrebinko, R.L., & Nelson, J.B. (2001). The treatment of prostate cancer: An overview of current options. *Cancer Practice, 9*(6), 295–306.

Pollack, A., Zagars, G.K., Starkschall, G., Antolak, J.A., Lee, J.J., Huang, E., et al. (2002). Prostate cancer radiation dose response: Results of the M.D. Anderson Phase III Randomized Trial. *International Journal of Radiation Oncology, Biology, Physics, 53*(5), 1097–1105.

Pomerantz, M., Manola, J., Taplin, M., Bubley, G., Inman, M., Lowell, J., et al. (2007). Phase II study of low dose and high dose conjugated estrogen for androgen independent prostate cancer. *Journal of Urology, 177*(6), 2146–2150.

Potosky, A.L., Davis, W.W., Hoffman, R.M., Stanford, J.L., Stephenson, R.A., Penson, D.F., et al. (2004). Five-year outcomes after prostatectomy or radiotherapy for prostate cancer. *Journal of the National Cancer Institute, 96*(18), 1358–1367.

Potters, L., Klein, E.A., Kattan, M.W., Reddy, C.A., Ciezki, J.P., Reuther, A.M., et al. (2004). Monotherapy for stage T1-T2 prostate cancer: Radical prostatectomy, external beam radiotherapy, or permanent seed implantation. *Radiotherapy and Oncology, 71*(1), 29–33.

Pu, X.Y., Wang, X.H., Wu, Y.L., & Wang, H.P. (2007). Comparative study of the impact of 3- versus 8-month neoadjuvant hormonal therapy on outcome of laparoscopic radical prostatectomy. *Journal of Cancer Research and Clinical Oncology, 133*(8), 555–562.

Ramsey, C.R., Scaperoth, D., Seibert, R., Chase, D., Byrne, T., & Mahan, S. (2007). Image-guided helical tomotherapy for localized prostate cancer: Technique and initial clinical observations. *Journal of Applied Clinical Medical Physics, 8*(3), 2320–2330.

Resche, I., Chatal, J.F., Pecking, A., Ell, P., Duchesne, G., Rubens, R., et al. (1997). A dose-controlled study of 153 Sm-Ethylenediaminetetramethylenephosphonate (EDTMP) in the treatment of patients with painful bone metastases. *European Journal of Cancer, 33*(10), 1583–1591.

Saad, F., Gleason, D.M., Murray, R., Tchekmedyian, S., Venner, P., Lacombe, L., et al. (2002). A randomized, placebo-controlled trial of zoledronic acid in patients with hormone-refractory metastatic prostate carcinoma. *Journal of the National Cancer Institute, 94*(19), 1458–1468.

Shelley, M., Harrison, G., Coles, B., Staffurth, J., Wilt, T.J., & Mason, M.D. (2006). Chemotherapy for hormone-refractory prostate cancer. *Cochrane Database of Systematic Reviews* 2006, Issue 4. Art. No.: CD005247. DOI: 10.1002/14651858.CD005247.pub2.

Schroder, F.H. (1998). Endocrine treatment of prostate cancer. In P.C. Walsh, A.B. Retik, E.D. Vaughan, & A.J. Wein (Eds.), *Campbell's urology* (7th ed., pp. 2627–2644). Philadelphia: Saunders.

Serber, W., Brady, L.W., Zhang, M., & Hoppe, R.T. (2004). Radiation treatment of benign disease. In C.A. Perez, L.W. Brady, E.C. Halperin, & R.K. Schmidt-Ullrich (Eds.), *Principles and practice of radiation oncology* (4th ed., pp. 2332–2351). Philadelphia: Lippincott Williams & Wilkins.

Sivalingam, S., Oxley, J., Probert, J.L., Stolzenburg, J.U., & Schwaibold, H. (2007). Role of pelvic lymphadenectomy in prostate cancer management. *Urology, 69*(2), 203–209.

Storlie, J.A., Buckner, J.C., Wiseman, G.A., Burch, P.A., Hartmann, L.C., & Richardson, R.L. (1995). Prostate specific antigen levels and clinical response to low dose dexamethasone for hormone-refractory metastatic prostate carcinoma. *Cancer, 76*(1), 96–100.

Sylvester, J.E., Blasko, J.C., Grimm, P.D., Meier, R., & Malmgren, J.A. (2003). Ten-year biochemical relapse-free survival after external beam radiation and brachytherapy for localized prostate cancer: The Seattle experience. *International Journal of Radiation Oncology, Biology, Physics, 57*(4), 944–952.

Tannock, I.F., de Wit, R., Berry, W.R., Horti, J., Pluzanska, A., Chi, K.N., et al. (2004). Docetaxel plus prednisone or mitoxantrone plus prednisone for advanced prostate cancer. *New England Journal of Medicine, 351*(15), 1502–1512.

Tannock, I.F., Osoba, D., Stockler, M.R., Ernst, D.S., Neville, A.J., Moore, M.J., et al. (1996). Chemotherapy with mitoxantrone and prednisone or prednisone alone for symptomatic hormone resistant prostate cancer: A Canadian randomized trial with palliative end points. *Journal of Clinical Oncology, 14*(6), 1756–1769.

Tannock, I., Gospodarowicz, M., Meakin, W., Panzarella, T., Stewart, L., & Rider, W. (1989). Treatment of metastatic prostatic cancer with low-dose prednisone evaluation of pain and quality of life as pragmatic indices of response. *Journal of Clinical Oncology, 7*(5), 590-597.

Temple, S.V. (2007). Radiopharmaceuticals. In M.L. Hass, W.P. Hogle, G.J. Moore-Higgs, & T.K. Gosselin-Acomb (Eds.), *Radiation therapy: A guide to patient care* (pp. 399–412). Philadelphia: Mosby.

Thompson, I., Thrasher, J.B., Aus, G., Burnett, A.L., Canby-Hagino, E.D., Cookson, M.S., et al. (2007). Guideline for the management of clinically localized prostate cancer: 2007 update. *Journal of Urology, 177*(6), 2106–2131.

Trofimov, A., Nguyen, P.L., Coen, J.J., Doppke, K.P., Schniefder, R., Adams, J.A., et al. (2007). Radiotherapy treatment of early-stage prostate cancer with IMRT and protons: A treatment planning comparison. *International Journal of Radiation Oncology, Biology, Physics, 69*(2), 444–453.

Vargas, C., Fryer, A., Mahajan, C., Indelicato, D., Horne, D., Chellini, A., et al. (2008). Dose-volume comparison of proton therapy and intensity-modulated radiotherapy for prostate cancer. *International Journal of Radiation Oncology, Biology, Physics, 70*(3), 744–751.

Verhey, L.J., & Munzenrider, J.E. (1982). Proton beam therapy. *Annual Review of Biophysics and Bioengineering, 11,* 331–357.

Zapatero, A., Rios, P., Marin, A., Minguez, R., & Garcia-Vecente, R. (2006). Dose escalation with three-dimensional conformal radiotherapy for prostate cancer. Is more dose really better in high-risk patients treated with androgen deprivation? *Clinical Oncology, 18*(8), 600–607.

Zelefsky, M.J., Valicenti, R.K., Goodman, K., & Perez, C.A. (2004). Male genitourinary tumors. In C.A. Perez, L.W. Brady, E.C. Halperin, & R.K. Schmidt-Ullrich (Eds.), *Principles and practice of radiation oncology* (4th ed., pp. 1692–1762). Philadelphia: Lippincott Williams & Wilkins.

Zietman, A.L., DeSilvio, M.L., Slater, J.D., Rossi, C.J., Miller, D.W., Adams, J.A., et al. (2005). Comparison of conventional-dose vs high-dose conformal radiation therapy in clinically localized adenocarcinoma of the prostate. *JAMA, 294*(10), 1233–1239.

CHAPTER 5

Nursing Implications of Prostate Cancer

Susan Moore, RN, MSN, ANP, AOCN®

Introduction

As previously noted, prostate cancer, one of the few gender-specific cancers, is the most common noncutaneous cancer among men. Prostate cancer is predominantly a tumor of older men, with a median age at diagnosis of 72 years (National Cancer Institute [NCI], 2007c). The growth rate of prostate cancer is highly variable, and older patients with localized disease may die of other illnesses without ever experiencing symptoms of prostate cancer. Three standard approaches exist for treating early prostate cancer: surgical removal of the prostate gland with or without lymph node sampling, radiation therapy (RT) with or without hormonal deprivation therapy, and watchful waiting or active surveillance. Hormonal therapy and systemic chemotherapy traditionally have been reserved for men with locally advanced or metastatic prostate cancer, although new applications of hormonal therapy as adjuncts to surgery or radiation show promise. Age and comorbid conditions influence treatment approach. Side effects of the various forms of treatment and patient preference should be considered in selecting the appropriate management of the disease. The best therapy is one that has been tailored to the individual needs and preferences of the patient and partner—one in which they clearly understand the risks and benefits and have made an active, informed decision to proceed with treatment.

Making a treatment choice is a high-risk decision involving critical thinking. Although treatment for many cancers is based on accumulated evidence from randomized, prospective clinical trials, data from phase III randomized, controlled clinical trials evaluating one prostate cancer treatment over another are lacking. Decisions can be made deliberately or by default when health conditions or age may limit options. Deliberate choices involve serious consideration of each treatment option and related side effects and effect on quality of life (QOL). Decision making can be a cause of anxiety and disruption in QOL for all involved in medical decisions. Maliski, Heilemann, and McCorkle (2002) found that couples made prostate cancer medical treatment decisions by each

spouse seeking information and then jointly discussing the options, leaving the final decision to the man. Davison et al. (2002) found that spouses preferred to play a collaborative role, leaving husbands in control of making the final decision regarding treatment choices. A nurse-run research study at the University of Washington (Personal Patient Profile–Prostate [P4]: A Randomized, Multi-Site Trial) seeks to determine whether participation in the P4 program is useful to men who are faced with choices about treatment for early-stage prostate cancer. The P4 program consists of a series of computer-based questions with printed and on-screen information for the participant. Participants access the P4 information before seeing the cancer specialist. Follow-up questionnaires are sent to the patient in the mail one month and six months after enrollment in the P4 program (Berry, 2007).

This chapter will address nursing implications of the following treatment options for localized and advanced prostate cancer.

- Watchful waiting, also called active surveillance or expectant management
- Hormonal manipulation
- Surgery
- Chemotherapy
- RT
- Radiopharmaceuticals

Watchful Waiting/Active Surveillance/ Expectant Management

Warlick, Trock, Landis, Epstein, and Carter (2006) studied the timing of surgical intervention in patients with small, lower-grade tumors in a small cohort of 38 patients who underwent delayed surgery versus 150 men who underwent immediate surgical intervention. Results showed that delayed prostate cancer surgery in patients with small, lower-grade prostate cancers did not appear to compromise curability. Men diagnosed with early-stage, lower-grade prostate cancer should not be led to believe that they have an urgent situation that requires immediate treatment. Warlick et al.'s data suggest that an expectant management approach should be used more frequently, given that approximately 50% of men today are diagnosed with low-risk prostate cancer.

The option of delaying prostate cancer treatment in early-stage, indolent, or asymptomatic disease in men who may be unable to tolerate aggressive therapy historically has been called *watchful waiting*. Recent publications have begun to use the terms *active surveillance* or *expectant management*. The new terms reflect a more positive approach. The goal of active surveillance is to spare patients with clinically localized disease the morbidity and mortality associated with more aggressive therapies (Griffin & O'Rourke, 2001). The first action during the initial treatment planning visit is to assess the probability that a given patient's prostate cancer poses a threat to survival and whether treatment is indicated at all. Active surveillance is a reasonable option in men who, based on their tumor-specific variables, age, comorbid conditions, and overall health, have a low risk of mortality from prostate cancer. Principles of active surveillance in prostate cancer management are available online from the National Comprehensive Cancer Network (NCCN, 2008) and are listed in Chapter 4 (see Figure 4-1). Patients in active surveillance generally are seen by the urologist or medical oncologist every six months with review of systems, prostate-specific antigen (PSA) testing, and a digital rectal examination performed at each visit to monitor the disease.

During active surveillance, the nurse needs to recognize that this is a time of great uncertainty and anxiety for the patient, partner, and family. The lack of formal guidelines to direct care during active surveillance may lead to patient anxiety. Patients may perceive this period as "doing nothing" or "not knowing." Patient strategies to relieve emotional distress include participating in a support group, praying (Walton & Sullivan, 2004), taking nutritional supplements reported to improve prostate health, and information seeking via the Internet (Griffin & O'Rourke, 2001). Men with prostate cancer often are advised to make changes in diet and lifestyle, but the impact of these changes previously had not been well documented. Ornish et al. (2005) evaluated the effects of comprehensive lifestyle changes on PSA level and serum-stimulated LNCaP (a line of androgen-sensitive human prostate cancer cells used in laboratory studies [produced by American Type Culture Collection]) cell growth in men with early, biopsy-proven prostate cancer after one year. PSA decreased 4% in the experimental group but increased 6% in the control group (p = .016). The growth of LNCaP prostate cancer cells was inhibited almost eightfold by serum from the experimental group compared to the control group (70% versus 9%, p < .001). Changes in serum PSA and in LNCaP cell growth were significantly associated with the degree of change in diet and lifestyle.

Patients and their partners may have different needs and coping mechanisms, and nurses must be prepared to work with each person separately as well as jointly (Giarelli, McCorkle, & Monturo, 2003; Northouse et al., 2007). Recognizing each patient's triggers for anxiety during active surveillance will help nurses to initiate patient and partner discussions about their concerns and provide reassurance regarding management strategies.

Hormonal Manipulation

Androgen deprivation therapy (ADT) is the mainstay treatment for prostate cancer, which is a hormonally driven cancer. ADT has been used to manage prostate cancer for decades, but current trends are to use ADT in earlier stages of disease. Hormones can be used as monotherapy or in combination with surgery or RT. Although most patients with metastatic disease receive continuous ADT, Tunn (2007) reported on the use of intermittent ADT, stating that preliminary support exists for equivalency of the two regimens, with improved QOL in the intermittent group. Bruchovsky, Klotz, Crook, and Goldenberg (2007) studied intermittent ADT in a prospective phase II trial for recurrent prostate cancer after radiotherapy and concluded that the length of the off-treatment interval during cyclic ADT was inversely related to baseline and nadir levels of serum PSA. Further consideration of intermittent ADT awaits the results of two large randomized clinical trials.

Assessment

A baseline physical examination and review of systems is necessary to determine patients' general health status before beginning ADT. Because some ADT agents may cause mild blood dyscrasias, baseline complete blood count (CBC) and liver function tests (LFTs) should be drawn before beginning therapy and monitored at regular intervals during treatment. Bone loss will occur during ADT (Guise, 2006; Shahinian, Kuo, Freeman, & Goodwin, 2005); therefore, a baseline dual-energy x-ray absorptiometry (DEXA) scan should be performed to evaluate bone density, as many older men may have already experienced a decrease in bone density caused by aging or poor diet.

Fertility options must be discussed with men who still desire to father children. Radical prostatectomy results in seminal fluid moving upward into the bladder instead of downward into the urethra, which prevents sperm from entering the ejaculate and results in sterility. ADT, RT, and cytotoxic chemotherapy commonly result in sterility, as well. Men facing therapy for prostate cancer may wish to consider sperm banking before undergoing surgery or other therapies (Ficorelli & Weeks, 2006).

Two recent large studies have documented a positive association between ADT and an increased incidence of diabetes, coronary heart disease, myocardial infarction (MI), and sudden cardiac death in men receiving gonadotropin-releasing hormone (GnRH) agonists (D'Amico et al., 2007; Keating, O'Malley, & Smith, 2006). Keating et al. analyzed Surveillance, Epidemiology, and End Results (SEER) data of 73,196 men age 66 and older and reported an increased risk (hazard ratios) for diabetes, 1.44; coronary heart disease, 1.16; MI, 1.11; and sudden cardiac death, 1.16. An unexpected finding was an increased risk of diabetes and coronary artery disease (CAD) in men on GnRH agonist therapy for as few as one to four months. The use of ADT has been associated with earlier onset of fatal MI in men age 65 and older who are treated with ADT for six to eight months when compared with men who did not receive ADT therapy or men younger than 65 years old (D'Amico et al.). The mechanism for this effect remains unknown. The authors of these studies recommend that men of advanced age planning to undergo ADT for prostate cancer should have a cardiovascular evaluation before the initiation of ADT. If clinically significant CAD is identified, then risk factor modification, appropriate pharmacologic interventions, and mechanical interventions should be considered before initiating ADT (D'Amico et al.; Keating et al.).

Symptom Management

Because hormonal therapy blocks testosterone, ADT can cause a number of distressing side effects similar to menopause in females. The side effects vary depending on the type of hormones and the length of time for which they are given. Common side effects include hot flashes, decreased libido (loss of or decreased sex drive), impotence (inability to have erections or successful intercourse), bone loss, and gynecomastia (breast enlargement). Hormones may also cause mild neutropenia, anemia, or elevation of liver enzymes. Some patients on hormones also complain of fatigue, arthralgia, or myalgia.

Hot Flashes

Hot flashes are a common complaint of both men and women on hormonal therapy for cancer, and the management in both sexes is essentially the same. Approximately 80% of men on ADT for prostate cancer will experience hot flashes (Kagee, Kruus, Malkowicz, Vaughn, & Coyne, 2001; Moore, 2004). Changes in lifestyle and environment may help to relieve mild hot flashes. Avoiding alcohol, caffeine, and highly spiced foods, maintaining cool room temperatures, and avoiding heavy sleepwear and bedding may provide some relief. Dressing in layers is recommended so that clothing can be removed easily during a hot flash. Nonpharmacologic approaches to hot flash management include herbal products derived from the more than 300 plants known to contain phytoestrogenic compounds. Soy isoflavones are the best-known source of phytoestrogens. *Cimicifuga racemosa*, commonly known as black cohosh, does not contain phytoestrogen but is reported in consumer literature to alleviate hot flashes. The

U.S. Food and Drug Administration (FDA) does not regulate food or herbal products, and the limited number of clinical trials evaluating these products does little to resolve issues of efficacy and safety (Moore). Most clinicians discourage the use of alternative therapies in the absence of large phase III randomized, placebo-controlled studies. Whether the efficacy and safety of any of these products in the breast cancer population can be generalized to other cancer populations, such as prostate cancer, remains to be supported by large-scale clinical trials.

Pharmacologic management includes the use of selective serotonin reuptake inhibitors (SSRIs) and antiseizure medications, interventions that have been widely studied in breast cancer survivors with treatment-related hot flashes. The SSRIs venlafaxine, fluoxetine, and paroxetine have been shown to be effective (Moore, 2004; Thompson, Shanafelt, & Loprinzi, 2003), as has gabapentin, an antiseizure medication (Loprinzi et al., 2007). A placebo-controlled, phase III multicenter clinical trial, NCT00354432, is comparing soy and venlafaxine alone or in combination for hot flash management in men receiving ADT for prostate cancer and currently is accruing patients (NCI, 2007a). Fewer than half of patients with prostate cancer on ADT experiencing discomfort during hot flashes stated that they would consider taking medication to relieve their symptoms (Kagee et al., 2001).

Gynecomastia

Gynecomastia (enlargement of the male glandular breast tissue) is a relatively common idiopathic disorder in the older adult male population. In prostate cancer ADT clinical trials, the incidence of gynecomastia ranged from 14%–71%, although the exact incidence is difficult to determine in short-term clinical trials because gynecomastia often appears six months or later after therapy (Dobs & Darkes, 2005). In a study of bicalutamide added to standard care (surgery, RT, or active surveillance), gynecomastia occurred in 68.8% of bicalutamide-treated patients and in 8.3% of placebo patients (McLeod et al., 2006). Breast pain and gynecomastia were mild or moderate in more than 90% of cases (Dobs & Darkes; Wirth et al., 2006). Gynecomastia has a physically and mentally deleterious effect on men, who may become self-conscious and embarrassed. It decreases QOL by causing physical pain and emotional discomfort and by disrupting lifestyles (Dobs & Darkes).

The etiology of gynecomastia ranges from benign physiologic processes to rare neoplasms, such as breast or pituitary cancers. Parallel to female breast development, estrogen, along with growth hormone and insulin-like growth factor-1, is required for breast growth in males. Because a balance exists between estrogen and androgens in males, any disease state or medication that increases circulating estrogen or decreases circulating androgen, causing an elevation in the estrogen-to-androgen ratio, can induce gynecomastia (Dobs & Darkes, 2005). Gynecomastia is more likely to occur with antiandrogen therapy or combination antiandrogen and ADT than with ADT monotherapy (See et al., 2002).

The most frequent clinical presentation of gynecomastia is localized breast pain or tenderness and patient- or partner-observed increased breast mass. The anatomic presentation of gynecomastia generally is symmetrical. It is important to establish that the patient has treatment-associated gynecomastia and to identify potential complicating conditions (concomitant medications and comorbid conditions) that may influence management. A thorough history should be obtained, including patient age, duration and onset of breast enlargement, symptoms of pain or tenderness, and concomitant medical or recreational drug use. The clinician should specifically evaluate the patient for potential breast malignancy, typically manifesting as a breast mass or focal tenderness. If a unilateral abnormality or a firm, hard lump is found, especially in the presence of a family history of breast cancer, a mammogram and further work-up, including biopsy, are required (Dobs & Darkes, 2005).

Gynecomastia can be graded according to the Common Terminology Criteria for Adverse Events (CTCAE) version 3.0 (NCI Cancer Therapy Evaluation Program, 2006) or the Simon classification (Simon, Hoffman, & Kahn, 1973). Table 5-1 compares the CTCAE grades and Simon classification. If no underlying pathology is discovered and the patient is on ADT, gynecomastia can be presumed to be caused by ADT, and observation is appropriate for mild or moderate cases. When gynecomastia is severe or distressing in patients who require continued hormonal therapy, medical therapy can be attempted, and if ineffective, glandular tissue can be removed surgically (Dobs & Darkes, 2005).

Tamoxifen, an estrogen antagonist, is effective for recent-onset and tender gynecomastia when given in doses of 10–20 mg twice a day. Up to 80% of patients report partial to complete resolution. Tamoxifen typically is tried for three months before the patient is referred to a surgeon (Boccardo et al., 2005). Perdona et al. (2005) reported the results of a phase III trial of tamoxifen in patients with prostate cancer who were taking bicalutamide. Investigators randomly assigned patients to 150 mg bicalutamide per day; 150 mg bicalutamide per day plus 10 mg tamoxifen per day for 24 weeks; and 150 mg bicalutamide per day plus RT (one 12 gray [Gy] fraction on day one of bicalutamide therapy). Results showed that 69% of patients on bicalutamide monotherapy developed gynecomastia, compared with 8% of those assigned to bicalutamide and tamoxifen, and 34% of those assigned to bicalutamide and RT. More than half of the patients on bicalutamide monotherapy experienced breast pain, compared with 6% of the patients on bicalutamide and tamoxifen, and 30% of the patients on bicalutamide and RT.

Low-dose prophylactic irradiation has been reported to reduce the rate of gynecomastia in men receiving estrogens or antiandrogens for advanced prostate cancer. Radiation dosage typically ranges from 12–15 Gy given over three to four fractions (treatments) (Serber, Brady, Zhang, & Hoppe, 2004). One side effect of irradiation is increased fibrosis of the tissue, thus making subsequent use of liposuction difficult should breast enlargement occur after radiation (Perdona et al., 2005; Prezioso et al., 2004; Widmark et al., 2003). If surgical correction is indicated or desired by the patient, low-grade gynecomastia is best treated early with liposuction alone because of increasing fibrosis as gynecomastia progresses (Prezioso et al.). Liposuction is performed on an outpatient basis, and the patient must wear a compression vest for a month while the chest wall heals (Nakabayashi, Bartlett, & Oh, 2006; Tashkandi, Al-Qattan, Hassanain, Hawary, & Sultan, 2004). Surgical management of high-grade gynecomastia (Simon grade III) has remained problematic because both liposuction and conventional subcutaneous mastectomy (without skin excision) frequently have resulted in significant residual skin redundancy, requiring a second operation for skin resection. One approach to high-grade gynecomastia has been single-stage subcutaneous mastectomy and circumareolar concentric skin reduction with de-epithelialization. This procedure, similar to reduction mammoplasty, removes excess skin and reshapes the chest (Tashkandi et al.). Insurance generally does not cover male breast reduction, and costs often exceed $6,000 (Nakabayashi et al.; Tashkandi et al.).

Arthralgia and Myalgia

ADT can cause significant symptoms of joint pain (arthralgia) and diffuse muscle pain, usually accompanied by malaise (myalgia) (Martin, 2004). A thorough history and physical examination with a focus on pain assessment (timing of onset, duration, location, severity, character, interventions, and response) and concomitant medications, activities, and self-treatment are the first steps in assessment. Most important is the character of the pain, which will help to differentiate neurotoxicity secondary to taxanes or diabetes from musculoskeletal pain associated with other causes. Functional assessment may also help in narrowing differential diagnoses. Concomitant drugs may provide clues (e.g., myopathy is a common side effect of corticosteroids used in prostate cancer treatment and for other concurrent conditions). Withdrawal from corticosteroids may cause a rheumatologic syndrome that includes arthralgia and myalgia (Martin). No specific diagnostic tests exist for arthralgia or mylagia; the diagnosis is one of exclusion based on physical examination and history.

The pathogenesis of arthralgia and myalgia secondary to ADT remains unclear; therefore, no specific treatment is available. Management of arthralgia and myalgia involves patient recognition of the signs of these conditions and continuing reassessment to evaluate the efficacy of interventions. Nonpharmacologic interventions include mild exercise, hydrotherapy, relaxation therapy, application of heat, and massage. A variety of medications can be used in stepwise fashion to decrease symptoms. Despite the fact that steroids can be a cause of arthralgia and myalgia, use of intermittent

Table 5-1. Gynecomastia: Comparison of Common Terminology Criteria for Adverse Events (CTCAE) Grades and Simon Classification

Grade	CTCAE Grading	Simon Classification
I	None	Small breast enlargement with localized button of tissue that is concentrated around the areola
II	Asymptomatic breast enlargement	Moderate breast enlargement exceeding areola boundaries with edges that are indistinct from the chest
III	Symptomatic breast enlargement; intervention indicated	Moderate breast enlargement exceeding areola boundaries with edges that are distinct from the chest with skin redundancy present
IV	Not applicable	Marked breast enlargement with skin redundancy and feminization of the breast

Note. Based on information from National Cancer Institute Cancer Therapy Evaluation Program, 2006; Simon et al., 1973.

steroids as well as nonsteroidal anti-inflammatory drugs (NSAIDs) can control discomfort. Both drug classes have anti-inflammatory properties, and NSAIDs also provide analgesic benefit (Martin, 2004).

Testosterone Surge and Flare Reaction

GnRH agonist treatment is well known to initially cause a testosterone surge and flare reaction resulting in moderate to severe bone pain in patients with metastatic prostate cancer. This is because of acute stimulation of prostate cancer cell growth by elevated levels of testosterone. A placebo-controlled trial has shown that antiandrogen therapy lowers the amount of bone pain with initiation of GnRH agonist therapy in patients with metastatic prostate cancer (Sharifi, Gulley, & Dahut, 2005). To prevent flare reactions, NCCN guidelines recommend that patients with metastatic disease start with an antiandrogen prior to initiation of treatment with a GnRH agonist and continue the antiandrogen for two to four weeks to block the effect of the testosterone surge on peripheral androgen receptors (NCCN, 2008).

Surgery

Surgical options for management of localized prostate cancer include radical retropubic prostatectomy, radical perineal prostatectomy, laparoscopic radical prostatectomy, or robot-assisted laparoscopic radical prostatectomy. Transurethral resection of the prostate (TURP) is palliative, not curative, and is performed to relieve symptoms such as urinary obstruction in patients with advanced prostate cancer or to treat benign prostatic hyperplasia and will not be discussed in detail in this chapter. Orchiectomy is surgical removal of the testes resulting in surgical castration and is considered an alternative to hormonal treatment. Orchiectomy does not remove the prostate gland itself; this procedure is used as a means of hormonal ablation to control prostate cancer. Since the advent of injectable GnRH agonists and nonsteroidal an-

tiandrogens, surgical castration is no longer favored (Potosky et al., 2002). Cryosurgery applies intense cold through a probe to destroy tumors by alternately freezing and thawing tissue. No long-term studies exist that compare cryosurgery to either RT or standard surgery to prove its effectiveness. Cryosurgery may be used in patients with locally recurrent prostate cancer who are not candidates for other forms of local treatment. Recent studies reported incontinence rates of 1.3%–7.5% and 6.7%–11% for primary and salvage cases, respectively (Ahmed, Lindsey, & Davies, 2005; Han & Belldegrun, 2004). Patients with a history of TURP may be at greater risk for incontinence after cryosurgery. Erectile dysfunction (ED) is the most common complication of cryosurgery, with most studies reporting greater than 70% incidence, although late recovery has been reported (Ahmed & Davies, 2005). The incidence of rectourethral fistula is reported at 0.5% (Han & Belldegrun).

Assessment

Assessment of the patient throughout the surgical continuum is important to decrease mortality and morbidity and ensure quality outcomes. Preoperatively, a complete physical examination should be performed along with a thorough medical and surgical history, medications (including vitamins and herbals), and any prior adverse reactions to anesthesia or delayed surgical recovery. A thorough history of preexisting pain related to cancer and comorbidities, such as arthritis, neuropathy, or other conditions, also should be obtained. This is an ideal time for the clinician to teach the patient how to report pain using the 0–10 pain scale, which will be used throughout the cancer continuum. Routine laboratory testing should be performed, either by the surgeon or by the patient's primary care provider. Any abnormal findings should be thoroughly evaluated before clearing the patient for surgery. Alibhai et al. (2005) conducted a retrospective chart review of more than 11,000 men who underwent radical prostatectomy from 1990–1999. They found that increasing comorbidity is a stronger predictor than age for almost all categories of early complications following radical prostatectomy and concluded that the risk of postoperative mortality after radical prostatectomy is relatively low for otherwise healthy older men up to age 79 (0.66%; 95% confidence interval [CI] = 0.2%–1.1%).

Preoperative Assessment

The goal of preoperative assessment is to identify potential problems that contribute to surgical morbidity and develop a plan to return patients to presurgical function as rapidly as possible (Barnett, 2005). Oncology nurse practitioners (ONPs) have an active role in the complex needs of preoperative patients by assuming responsibility for preoperative physical assessment, ordering necessary laboratory tests or procedures, providing referral for consultation as needed, and documenting medical clearance for surgery. ONPs recognize the medical, educational, and emotional issues that men face related to undergoing prostatectomy. Patients who are properly prepared for surgery have a more positive perioperative experience (Barnett).

Preoperative assessment of older adult patients with prostate cancer is essential to ensure that surgery is performed only on those patients who are likely to benefit from surgical intervention and are physically able to tolerate the procedure. Assessment scales may supplement physical exam and also plan for postoperative resource allocation. The Physiological and Operative Severity Score for the enUmeration of Mortality and morbidity (POSSUM) scale was specifically developed for patients undergoing surgery and includes 12 physiologic and 6 operative variables (Copeland, Jones, & Walters, 1991). POSSUM predicts morbidity and postoperative mortality in general surgery and in patients with lung cancer and colorectal cancer. Criticisms of POSSUM are that it uses complex data (although most of this physiologic information is available in the routine preoperative assessment of older adult patients) and that it has not been validated in prostate cancer. Anecdotally, the preoperative use of POSSUM appears to be increasing in prostate and other surgical procedures despite being outside the original validation of the system (Ramanathan, Moppett, Wenn, & Moran, 2005). POSSUM was designed as a postoperative, general surgical audit tool in 1991. Its use has expanded into specialty surgical fields and preoperative assessment. If it is to be used with confidence, POSSUM needs to be validated for specific surgical procedures. Although POSSUM provides some evidence of preoperative physiologic frailty, most data are provided in the immediate postoperative period. POSSUM may be useful in the preoperative selection of older adult patients and in the immediate postoperative prediction of morbidity and mortality (Gosney, 2005).

Preoperative teaching of the surgical patient and his partner must include a full discussion of the risks and benefits of each procedure, if a procedure choice is possible. The risks with orchiectomy or any radical prostatectomy approach are comparable to most major surgical procedures. Risks include heart attack, stroke, thromboembolic events, bleeding at the surgical site intra- and postoperatively, and adverse reactions to anesthesia. Possible side effects of radical prostatectomy are urinary incontinence and impotence. Penson et al. (2005) reported the five-year urinary and sexual outcomes from the Prostate Cancer Outcomes Study. A sample of 1,288 men treated with radical prostatectomy for localized prostate cancer were surveyed: 14% reported frequent urinary leakage or no urinary control 60 months after diagnosis, which was slightly higher than the 10% reporting incontinence at 24 months (p = .007). At 60 months, 28% of the men had erections firm enough for intercourse, compared with 22% at 24 months (p = .003). Incontinence and impotence are not restricted to surgical outcomes; they are potential side effects of other prostate cancer therapy modalities as well. Moore, Truong, Estey, and Voaklander (2007) studied incontinence at baseline and following radical prostatectomy. Preoperative risk factors affecting continence were increasing age, baseline incontinence, and previous TURP. Mean International Prostate Symptom Score was lower at 12 months than at baseline, suggesting that even mildly symptomatic men will improve after surgery.

Burt, Caelli, Moore, and Anderson (2005) reported on men's experiences after radical prostatectomy and whether they perceived that their preoperative teaching adequately prepared them for postoperative recovery. Although patients received verbal and written instruction about postoperative expectations and care before radical prostatectomy, they expressed concern about a lack of preparation in managing urinary incontinence and ED. Pre- and postoperative teaching needs to make allowances for the impact of stress on the recall and processing of information. Follow-up telephone support is recommended to support adjustment after surgery. This study showed that written information in itself is not adequate to answer necessary questions and provide reassurance; nurses need to be prepared, both educationally and psychologically, to observe nonverbal cues and to address questions and concerns that are rarely voiced in ways that indicate their significance to the person; and men may not speak about sexuality issues in ways that accurately reflect the extent of their worry or distress about ED (Burt et al.). Incontinence and ED, both common complications of treatment for prostate cancer, are discussed in a separate section of this chapter.

Postoperative Assessment

The postoperative period involves management of pain and return to normal functioning. A comprehensive postoperative physical evaluation with focus on the operative site, urinary output, respiratory and cardiac function, and pain level is imperative. Assessment of the surgical site for signs of infection or wound dehiscence should be done routinely, and any changes must be documented and reported promptly to the surgeon. All patients will have an indwelling urinary catheter in place after prostatectomy. Output should be monitored for amount and the appearance of blood or cloudy, foul-smelling urine.

Cancer pain can be caused by tumor or treatment. This section addresses pain caused by surgical resection for treatment of prostate cancer. Most postoperative pain is acute, which generally is defined as occurring during a period of less than three months (McGuire, 2004; Paice, 2004). A thorough history of preoperative pain should be part of the patient's record when being admitted to the postoperative setting, and complete pain assessment should be conducted with each new complaint of pain or when altering the treatment plan (Paice). Using a standard 0–10 pain scale for pain assessment, with 0 indicating no pain and 10 indicating the worst pain the patient could imagine, is standard policy in most institutions. Assessment and intervention for pain became an accreditation standard by the Joint Commission on the Accreditation of Healthcare Organizations in 2001 and was updated in 2004. Patients with dementia, delirium, or other disorders that preclude use of the 0–10 scale can be observed for facial expressions or altered behaviors as signs of pain (Snow & Shuster, 2006). Cancer pain management generally follows the analgesic pain relief ladder developed by the World Health Organization (WHO, 2007). Although designed for management of disease-related pain, the WHO ladder can be used for postoperative pain management as well. Adjunct medications such as tricyclic antidepressants, anticonvulsants, local anesthetics, and corticosteroids can be added to nonopioids and opioids as needed for full control of pain. Undesirable interactions caused by drugs such as antihistamines, benzodiazepines, antidepressants, and antipsychotic drugs can lead to increased sedation (Strassels, McNicol, & Suleman, 2005).

Symptom Management

Pain Management

An in-depth discussion of management of acute postoperative pain is outside the scope of this chapter. A wealth of evidence-based literature is available that addresses both cancer-related and postoperative pain syndromes. Interventions, whether pharmacologic or nonpharmacologic, must be individualized to the patient needs at each time point in the treatment continuum. The American Society of Anesthesiologists Task Force on Acute Pain Management (2004) published guidelines for the management of postoperative pain. Additional pain-related clinical practice guidelines and resources are available through professional and advocacy groups, including the American Pain Society and the Cochrane Collaboration (Strassels et al., 2005).

Management of Cryosurgery Complications

Complications of cryosurgery include urinary incontinence, ED, perineal pain, urethral sloughing, rectourethral fistula, and urethral/bladder neck stricture. Perineal pain occurs in up to 11% of patients having primary cryosurgery

but is more common when cryosurgery is performed after RT (Ahmed et al., 2005). Persistent perineal pain should be evaluated by cystoscopy and pelvic ultrasound to exclude urethral sloughing and abscess. Treatment with an NSAID and tepid sitz baths usually is sufficient, but more severe pain may require narcotics. Urethral sloughing results from necrosis of the prostatic urethra, may occur three to eight weeks following cryosurgery, and may be identified during work-up for perineal pain. Patients generally present with pain, pyuria, or urinary retention. Diagnosis is by cystoscopy. Urethral sloughing is treated by prolonged indwelling catheterization or intermittent self-catheterization. Persistent symptoms may require TURP for resolution. Although development of a rectourethral fistula is uncommon, patients who had prior RT are at increased risk. Most patients with a fistula present with watery diarrhea or stool in the urine (fecaluria), recurrent bladder infections, or sepsis. A voiding urethrogram, computed tomography, or magnetic resonance imaging will confirm the presence of a fistula. Conservative management includes antibiotics for infection or sepsis, insertion of a urinary catheter, and consultation with a wound, ostomy, and continence (WOC) nurse. Persistent fistulas may require surgical repair, preferably with a multidisciplinary team including a urologist, a colorectal surgeon, and a WOC nurse. Stricture of the urethral/bladder neck is the result of scar tissue formation and generally occurs in the presence of extensive tissue sloughing. The use of warming catheters during cryosurgery has virtually eliminated this complication; if it does occur, a transurethral incision or limited resection of scar tissue usually provides relief (Ahmed & Davies, 2005).

Postoperative Patient Education

At discharge, patients must be instructed on how to care for incision sites, dressings, and the indwelling urinary catheter. Pain medication schedules and management of breakthrough pain also must be clearly communicated to the patient and in-home caregivers to avoid unnecessary pain and anxiety. Informing patients about any expected side effects from surgery will lessen anxiety. Follow-up appointments with the urologist, surgeon, or medical oncologist should be scheduled before discharge, if possible, so that patients can arrange transportation and family member attendance.

After radical prostatectomy, detectable PSA levels may identify patients who are at elevated risk for local treatment failure or metastatic disease. However, a substantial proportion of patients with elevated or rising PSA levels after surgery may remain asymptomatic for extended periods of time. Biochemical failure (rising PSA after definitive treatment) alone may not be sufficient to alter treatment. For example, in a retrospective analysis of nearly 2,000 men who had undergone radical prostatectomy with curative intent and who were followed for a mean of 5.3 years, 315 (15%) demonstrated an abnormal PSA level of 0.2 ng/ml or higher, which is evidence of biochemical recurrence. Of these 315,

103 men (34%) developed clinical evidence of recurrence. The median time to development of clinical metastasis after biochemical recurrence was eight years. After the men developed metastatic disease, the median time to death was an additional five years (Pound et al., 1999).

Chemotherapy

The majority of men who undergo androgen deprivation, by means of either ADT or bilateral orchiectomy, eventually progress to an androgen-independent phase where the initial ADT regimen no longer controls the tumor (Diaz & Patterson, 2004; Gallagher & Gapstur, 2006). A minority of men who have progressive disease after initial ADT respond to additional hormonal treatments. Prostate cancer that no longer responds to any hormonal treatment is referred to as hormone-refractory prostate cancer (HRPC) (Diaz & Patterson). Historically, cytotoxic chemotherapy for prostate cancer induced low response rates (Penson, Chan, & Urologic Diseases in America Project, 2007). Prior to the use of taxanes, no survival benefit supporting the use of chemotherapy was demonstrated. More recent studies of chemotherapy in patients with HRPC report benefits including reduced pain, improved QOL, and decreased need for narcotics (Berthold, Sternberg, & Tannock, 2005; Petrylak et al., 2004). The choice between using chemotherapy or a secondary hormonal therapy when androgen withdrawal has failed is based on clinical judgment; few comparative studies are available (Sharifi et al., 2005).

Currently, only docetaxel, estramustine, and mitoxantrone have received FDA approval for the treatment of advanced prostate cancer, although other drugs such as paclitaxel, vinorelbine, and etoposide are used off-label. The survival benefit of docetaxel is modest—two to three months—and a large proportion of patients with HRPC become refractory to taxane-based treatment (Berthold et al., 2005). Recent publications suggest that docetaxel alone or combined with estramustine, with or without prednisone, may be the optimal treatment for HRPC (Eymard et al., 2007; Goodin et al., 2005). Two phase III clinical trials comparing docetaxel-based regimens to mitoxantrone-based regimens in HRPC reported superior survival and improved response in terms of pain, serum PSA level, and QOL in the docetaxel plus prednisone groups (Petrylak et al., 2004; Tannock et al., 2004). Docetaxel-based regimens currently are considered the standard of care in the treatment of HRPC (NCCN, 2008) and should be presented as a treatment option for patients with HRPC; however, patients should make an informed decision based on the overall risks and benefits of chemotherapy. Experience is limited with the use of chemotherapy in patients with hormone-sensitive disease. Results of a neoadjuvant study of a chemohormonal regimen (docetaxel plus estramustine) in nonmetastatic high-risk prostate cancer found that the neoadjuvant chemohormonal regimen is feasible and active in

patients with high-risk prostate cancer (Prayer-Galetti et al., 2007). Responding patients had an 85% disease-free survival rate at five years.

Estramustine, a combined estradiol derivative and alkylating agent, has activity in prostate cancer and can be administered intravenously or orally. The IV preparation is associated with superficial phlebitis and hepatotoxicity. The oral preparation is associated with nausea and vomiting, edema, deep vein thrombosis, and myelosuppression. Common side effects include breast tenderness and gynecomastia, decreased libido, and ED (Pfizer Inc., 2006a).

An investigational agent showing promise in HRPC is ixabepilone (BMS-247550), a semisynthetic derivative of epothilone B. Epothilone B and its analogs are a relatively new classification of antineoplastic agents and have a unique mode of tubulin binding that may make these drugs more likely to overcome taxane resistance (Dawson, 2007). In a phase II study reported by Hussain et al. (2004), the most frequent toxicities of ixabepilone were neutropenia, peripheral neuropathy, and fatigue. Another investigational agent, satraplatin, the first oral platinum analog, has been shown to improve disease-free survival in HRPC. The dose-limiting toxicity of satraplatin is myelosuppression, which is dose-dependent and reversible upon stopping the drug (Sternberg et al., 2005). Results of a phase III multinational placebo-controlled clinical trial of satraplatin plus prednisone versus placebo plus prednisone in HRPC showed a 33% increase in median progression-free survival in the satraplatin group (Sternberg et al., 2007). Other studies of combination regimens including angiogenesis inhibitors, endothelin axis blockers, small molecules, and antisense targets with docetaxel are under way at several institutions (NCI, 2007a).

Cytotoxic chemotherapy can cause widespread adverse effects because of the systemic nature of treatment. Specific side effects of antineoplastic agents commonly used for treatment of HRPC are detailed in Table 5-2. Table 5-3 outlines management of selected chemotherapy side effects. The FDA-approved agents for treatment of prostate cancer include docetaxel, estramustine, mitoxantrone, and prednisone.

Prechemotherapy Assessment

The overall condition of men about to undergo systemic chemotherapy for prostate cancer should be carefully evaluated before initiating therapy. General weakness and poor nutritional status and the inability to follow instructions regarding self-care during chemotherapy may increase the severity of side effects. Evaluation of these contributing factors should be part of the prechemotherapy assessment before making treatment decisions. The chronologic age of the patient should not preclude treatment, as age alone is not an accurate predictor of an individual's tolerance of aggressive therapy. With few exceptions, cancer treatment is as effective in older individuals as in the young; however, older people are

Table 5-2. Adverse Effects of Antineoplastic Agents and Supportive Drugs Commonly Used for Treatment of Prostate Cancer

Antineoplastic Agent/ Supportive Drug	Drug Classification	Method of Administration	Adverse Effects
Docetaxel	Taxane	IV	Neutropenia Peripheral neuropathy Nausea and vomiting Diarrhea Hypersensitivity reaction Peripheral edema Hyperglycemia (attributable to steroid premedication) Alopecia Hand-foot syndrome Paronychia Epiphora (excessive tearing) Canalicular stenosis (with weekly dosing)
Estramustine	Estradiol plus nor-nitrogen mustard (alkylating agent)	IV or PO	Dyspnea Elevated liver function tests (LFTs) Gynecomastia Congestive heart failure Thromboembolic events Thrombocytopenia Leg cramps Nausea and vomiting Diarrhea Flatulence Peripheral edema
Mitoxantrone	Antitumor antibiotic	IV	Myelosuppression Elevated LFTs Arrhythmias Congestive heart failure Nausea Anorexia Constipation Blue-green discoloration of urine and sclera for 1–2 days following treatment Alopecia Vesicant properties; thus, care should be taken to avoid extravasation during administration
Prednisone Dexamethasone	Steroid	PO	Hyperglycemia Weight gain Increased risk of infection Insomnia or restlessness Indigestion or stomach irritation Bruising Acneform skin rash

Note. Based on information from Camp-Sorrell, 2005; Esmaeli & Hortobagyi, 2001; Esmaeli et al., 2001; Pietrzak et al., 2006; Schulmeister, 2005.

more susceptible to treatment-related side effects (Balducci & Ershler, 2005). Advanced practice nurses (APNs) and nurse clinicians must recognize the heterogeneity of the older adult population in order to focus their assessments appropriately. Before a treatment plan is determined, assessment of older adult men's functional ability is important. A commonly used geriatric assessment tool is the Comprehensive Geriatric Assessment (CGA), a multidimensional, interdisciplinary

diagnostic process that identifies medical, functional, and psychosocial problems in older adults (Rao, Seo, & Cohen, 2004; Rubenstein, 2004). Ingram et al. (2002) studied the feasibility of a self-report CGA in an outpatient cancer center and found that the self-report methodology provided valid data in terms of functional status, health status, and QOL. Functional performance scores and dependency at home appeared to be independent predictive factors for toxicity, similar to depres-

Table 5-3. Management of Selected Adverse Effects of Antineoplastic Agents and Supportive Drugs Used to Treat Hormone-Refractory Prostate Cancer

Adverse Effect	Causal Agent	Comments	Suggested Interventions
Nausea and vomiting (N&V)	Docetaxel Estramustine Mitoxantrone	• Docetaxel and estramustine have very low (< 10%) potential for N&V. • Mitoxantrone has a moderate (30%–60%) potential for N&V. • Refractory vomiting: Assess electrolytes; administer IV fluids; assess concomitant medications and comorbidities.	Mild to moderate N&V • Prochlorperazine 10 mg PO every 4–6 hours Moderate to severe N&V • 5-HT$_3$ receptor antagonist or NK$_1$ receptor agonist • Prochlorperazine 10 mg PO every 4–6 hours for breakthrough nausea or vomiting
Diarrhea	Docetaxel Estramustine	• Refractory diarrhea: Take stool specimen; assess electrolytes; administer IV fluids; assess concomitant medications and comorbidities.	• Loperamide 4 mg at first watery stool, 2 mg every 4 hours until diarrhea stops; recommended for use < 24 hours with maximum dose of 16 mg over 24 hours. • Consider octreotide subcutaneously TID, with dose titrated to effect for refractory diarrhea after work-up for cause of refractory diarrhea.
Constipation	Mitoxantrone	• Monitor bowel movement frequency and consistency; contact doctor or RN if no bowel movement in 48 hours or if stool becomes hard or dry or requires straining to evacuate.	• Begin prophylactic stool softener at start of therapy. • Increase dietary fiber or add psyllium supplement to daily intake. • Increase PO fluids. • Increase activity if tolerated. • Prescribe laxative PRN.
Neurotoxicity • Peripheral neuropathy • Arthralgia/myalgia	Docetaxel	• Mild sensory peripheral neuropathy until cumulative dose of 600 mg/m^2, when disabling neuropathy can result • Arthralgia/myalgia occurs infrequently beginning 1–3 days after administration; duration is ≤ 4 days.	Sensory neuropathy • Consider pyridoxine (vitamin B$_6$). • Consider gabapentin 300 mg PO TID, increasing dose to effect. • Consider referral to occupational therapist. Arthralgia/myalgia • Begin prophylactic nonsteroidal anti-inflammatory drugs; continue for 4–5 days after treatment. • Encourage mild exercise (walking, yoga).
Hand-foot syndrome	Docetaxel	–	• Initiate liberal use of skin emollients, preferably those containing lanolin, beginning at first dose. • Use tepid water when possible. • Avoid immersing hands or feet in harsh chemicals or desiccating solutions. • Avoid repetitive actions that cause abrasion to hands or feet. • Report redness or pain in hands or feet immediately.
Nail changes • Hyperpigmentation • Paronychia • Onycholysis	Docetaxel	• Nail hyperpigmentation occurs more often in dark-skinned individuals. • Hyperpigmentation is more pronounced at base of nails. • Patient may confuse paronychia or onycholysis with fungal infection.	Hyperpigmentation • Use sunscreen with sun protection factor of 30, and avoid long sun exposure. • Reassure patient that hyperpigmentation is temporary. Paronychia or onycholysis • Protect nails from trauma or injury. • Keep nails trimmed closely. • Consider referral to podiatrist for nail care or removal.

(Continued on next page)

Table 5-3. Management of Selected Adverse Effects of Antineoplastic Agents and Supportive Drugs Used to Treat Hormone-Refractory Prostate Cancer *(Continued)*

Adverse Effect	Causal Agent	Comments	Suggested Interventions
Alopecia	Mitoxantrone	• Hair loss generally is rare and most likely is manifested by thinning rather than frank hair loss. • Hair thinning begins 3–4 weeks after first mitoxantrone dose. • Hair thinning also may be caused by male pattern balding or androgen deprivation therapy.	• Prepare patient for hair loss regarding the timing and severity. • Advise patient to obtain a wig before hair loss occurs, if desired. • Provide written order for "cranial prosthesis" for insurance.
Myelosuppression • Neutropenia • Anemia • Thrombocytopenia	Mitoxantrone Docetaxel Estramustine	• Thrombocytopenia is unlikely.	Febrile neutropenia • Administer granulocyte–colony-stimulating factor either daily (filgrastim) or per cycle (pegfilgrastim) following prescribing information. Anemia • Administer erythropoiesis-stimulating agent for documented anemia following prescribing information (weekly epoetin alfa or long-acting darbepoetin). Thrombocytopenia • Consider platelet transfusion for platelet count < 10,000–20,000 cells/mm³.
Peripheral edema	Docetaxel Estramustine	• Monitor edema. • If persistent, refractory, or accompanied by other signs of heart failure, assess cardiac function.	Docetaxel • Administer dexamethasone 8 mg PO BID starting one day prior to dosing and continuing for a total of three days.
Hyperglycemia	Dexamethasone Prednisone	• Hyperglycemia is caused by supportive drugs, not the chemotherapy.	• Monitor blood glucose regularly in all patients on steroids. • Refer nondiabetic patients who have high blood glucose levels before or during therapy to internist or endocrinologist for evaluation and management. • Instruct diabetic patients to test blood glucose more than once daily. • Consider supplementing oral diabetes medication with insulin in patients who show evidence of poor control during steroid therapy.
Hepatotoxicity	Estramustine Mitoxantrone	–	• Monitor liver enzymes during chemotherapy. • Instruct patient to avoid alcohol intake. • Avoid concomitant hepatotoxic drugs. • Consider dose reduction for drugs metabolized in liver.
Hypersensitivity reaction	Docetaxel	• Dexamethasone is used to prevent edema but may have a protective effect against hypersensitivity reaction. • Monitor patient during infusion for hypotension, rash, itching, dyspnea, or bronchospasm.	• Administer dexamethasone 8 mg PO BID starting one day prior to dosing and continuing for a total of three days.

(Continued on next page)

Table 5-3. Management of Selected Adverse Effects of Antineoplastic Agents and Supportive Drugs Used to Treat Hormone-Refractory Prostate Cancer (Continued)

Adverse Effect	Causal Agent	Comments	Suggested Interventions
Ocular changes • Epiphora • Canalicular stenosis (with weekly dosing)	Docetaxel	• Avoid weekly docetaxel dosing (increased incidence of canalicular stenosis with weekly versus every-three-week dosing). • Refer to ophthalmologist for assessment, diagnosis of canalicular stenosis, and insertion of tubes, if needed.	• Obtain baseline history from patient regarding dry eyes or excessive tearing. • Consider referral to ophthalmologist for evaluation and exam if baseline assessment is abnormal. • Assess for excess tearing at each cycle.
Cardiac toxicity • Arrhythmias • Congestive heart failure	Mitoxantrone Estramustine	• Refer to cardiologist before treatment if abnormal.	• Obtain baseline electrocardiogram before treatment. • Evaluate cardiac function at each visit. • Evaluate for edema, cough, and dyspnea. • Positive signs: Evaluate with chest x-ray, multigated acquisition (MUGA) scan, or echocardiogram. If MUGA result is < the lower limit of normal or is significantly decreased from baseline MUGA, hold drug and refer to cardiologist for work-up.

Note. Based on information from Camp-Sorrell, 2005; Dipaola et al., 2004; Esmaeli & Hortobagyi, 2001; Eymard et al., 2007; Gallagher & Gapstur, 2006; Immunex Corp., 2002; Katz, 2007a; Pfizer Inc., 2006a; Sanofi-Aventis, 2003.

sive symptoms and polypharmacy (Maas, Janssen-Heijnen, Olde Rikkert, & Machteld, 2007). The clinical impact of CGA in oncology decision making has not been validated in prospective, randomized clinical trials.

Docetaxel

Thorough and careful neurologic assessment is critical in patients receiving potentially neurotoxic agents such as docetaxel. The baseline assessment should include sensory function, motor function, gait, range of motion, cranial nerves, and reflexes (Camp-Sorrell, 2005). Canalicular stenosis generally presents as excessive tearing and has been reported as a side effect to docetaxel, although it occurs more frequently in weekly administration than in the every-three-week administration used in prostate cancer (Camp-Sorrell; Esmaeli & Hortobagyi, 2001; Esmaeli, Valero, Ahmadi, & Booser, 2001). An ophthalmologist may perform a baseline eye examination, including assessment for dry eye or other ocular conditions.

Estramustine

Estramustine assessment should include evaluation of hepatic function by drawing baseline LFTs, reviewing a current CBC with careful attention to the platelet count, and obtaining a history of any thromboembolic events, specifically stroke or CAD. Physical examination should note any peripheral edema and evidence of circulatory deficiencies indicative of vascular disorders in the lower extremities (e.g., varicose veins, signs of peripheral vascular disease, arterial insufficiency) (Camp-Sorrell, 2005; Pfizer Inc., 2006a).

Mitoxantrone

A CBC is essential to determine baseline neutrophil and hemoglobin levels, as is a chemistry panel to evaluate LFTs. A complete medical history with special attention to cardiac events should be obtained. Patients with a history of cardiac arrhythmias, MI, or CAD should have a baseline electrocardiogram and evaluation by a cardiologist before treatment. Patients who are to receive mitoxantrone should be instructed about the common side effects of nausea and vomiting, myelosuppression, fatigue, increased risk of infection, and blue-green discoloration of urine and sclera (Berthold et al., 2005; Camp-Sorrell, 2005; Tannock et al., 2004).

Corticosteroids

A common side effect of steroid administration is hyperglycemia. A baseline blood glucose or hemoglobin A1c test should be evaluated before patients begin steroid therapy. Regular evaluation of blood glucose levels through the course of cortirosteroid therapy should be scheduled, and patients with high blood glucose should be referred to their primary care provider or an endocrinologist for diabetes management. Clinicians should obtain a complete list of concomitant medications to evaluate for interactions or other steroids prescribed for conditions such as lupus, asthma, eczema, or other inflammatory conditions. Additional side effects of steroid therapy include increased risk of infection, insomnia or restlessness, indigestion or stomach irritation, bruising, and acneform skin rash (Camp-Sorrell, 2005).

A major oncology nursing role is assessing for psychosocial morbidity and social support in patients. In a longitudinal study of QOL and psychosocial status of patients and their partners, Northouse et al. (2007) noted that patients with advanced prostate cancer reported more social support when receiving chemotherapy treatment for HRPC than when receiving ADT. Questions about whether this increase in social support is attributable to greater evidence of fear on the part of the patient or partner, the poor prognosis of HRPC, or a spontaneous response of the social network remain unanswered. Siston et al. (2003) examined QOL after diagnosis of prostate cancer and before treatment initiation among minority men of lower socioeconomic status. At 12 months, decreases in disease-specific QOL persisted for patients with localized disease, but for patients with metastatic disease, disease-specific QOL appeared to return to near baseline (at diagnosis, before treatment initiation) function.

Chemotherapy Patient Education

The oncology nurse should take the opportunity to meet with all patients who are beginning a chemotherapy regimen and their partner or other family members to discuss the medication, how it is given, the treatment interval, and expected side effects. Topics are individualized according to the regimen, patient status, and the patient's learning ability. A baseline assessment of learning barriers and accommodations to overcome any barriers (e.g., speech, hearing, or vision barriers) will help to make this session less stressful for all parties involved. Among the topics that should be covered, regardless of the proposed regimen, are identification of early signs of side effects; prevention of side effects (e.g., hygiene, supportive care measures, medications); whom to call with questions or problems, including after-hours access; management of potentially serious side effects, such as fever, vomiting, pain, or bleeding; and excretion precautions. In terms of bodily waste, patients should be instructed to flush the toilet twice with the lid closed during the 48 hours after receiving chemotherapy (Polovich, White, & Kelleher, 2005).

Docetaxel
Docetaxel is administered IV, generally every three weeks. Premedication with an oral steroid (dexamethasone) twice daily for three days (day before, day of, and day after treatment) is required to prevent peripheral edema and possible hypersensitivity reaction. The package insert (Sanofi-Aventis, 2003) contains sample dexamethasone instruction labels and a patient education sheet concerning dexamethasone administration and side effects. Docetaxel patient education key points include
- Take the prescribed doses of dexamethasone, a steroid, before and after your docetaxel infusion. If you forget, call your oncologist or nurse for instructions.
- Report any of the following side effects to your oncologist or nurse immediately:
  - Difficulty breathing; closing of the throat; swelling of the lips, tongue, or face; or hives

- Extreme fatigue; easy bruising or bleeding
- Signs of infection: fever or chills.
- Other symptoms to report include
  - Redness in the tissue or along the vein; reactions near the site of administration
  - Abdominal pain, yellowing of the skin or eyes
  - Severe nausea, vomiting, diarrhea, or loss of appetite
  - Swelling of the feet, ankles, or abdomen
  - Difficulty breathing
  - Skin redness or peeling, primarily on the palms of the hands and soles of the feet
  - Burning or tingling sensations, or numbness in the hands or feet
  - Changes in the appearance of fingernails or toenails.

Estramustine
Estramustine can be administered orally or by IV. In addition to educating patients about the expected side effects of estramustine (see Table 5-2), instruction on proper adherence to the oral regimen is needed. Key education points for the patient on estramustine therapy should include the following (Pfizer Inc., 2006a).
- Eat small meals frequently to help to alleviate nausea.
- Do not take estramustine with milk or milk products because calcium-containing foods (milk or milk products) may inhibit optimal absorption of estramustine.
- Encourage patients to speak with the oncologist or nurse about the timing of ingesting calcium-containing compounds such as antacids and taking estramustine. Ideally, patients should be switched to another class of antacid, such as a proton-pump inhibitor, or advised to take calcium-containing antacids either two hours before or two hours after the estramustine dose.
- Estramustine must be kept refrigerated. When traveling, take along a small cooler with frozen gel-packs to keep the medication cool.
- Estramustine should be taken either one hour before meals on an empty stomach or two hours after meals. Take with a full glass of water.
- If a dose is missed, do not double up the next dose.
- Avoid prolonged sun exposure. If sun exposure is unavoidable, wear sunscreen and protective clothing (hat, sunglasses, long-sleeve shirt, and long pants).
- Report any chest or leg pain; swelling of the legs, hands, face, or abdomen; difficulty breathing, headache; weakness in the arms or legs; yellowing of the eyes or skin; severe nausea or vomiting; or persistent diarrhea.

Mitoxantrone
Mitoxantrone is given IV and may be administered with or without prednisone. Patient education for patients receiving mitoxantrone includes the following (Immunex Corp., 2002).
- Drink at least two to three quarts of fluid every 24 hours, unless you are instructed otherwise.

- Your urine will probably be green or blue for one to two days after chemotherapy. Do not be concerned—this does not mean anything is wrong.
- When your white blood cell count is low, you may be at risk for infection. Avoid crowds or people with colds and those who are not feeling well.
- Report fever or any other signs of infection immediately to your oncologist or nurse.
- Wash your hands often.
- Use a soft toothbrush, and rinse your mouth three times a day with one-half to one teaspoon of baking soda and/or one-half to one teaspoon of salt mixed with 8 ounces of water, or an alcohol-free mouth rinse.
- Use an electric razor to minimize bleeding.
- Avoid contact sports or activities that could cause injury.
- Take antinausea medications as prescribed by your doctor or nurse.
- Eat small, frequent meals.
- Avoid prolonged sun exposure. If sun exposure is unavoidable, wear sunscreen and protective clothing (hat, sunglasses, long-sleeve shirt, and long pants).
- Avoid drinking alcoholic beverages completely or keep consumption to a minimum.

Corticosteroids

Oral prednisone, a corticosteroid, is an integral part of several chemotherapy regimens used in the treatment of advanced prostate cancer. Dexamethasone, a corticosteroid used during docetaxel therapy to prevent edema, requires similar patient education. Because patients will self-administer prednisone at home, they should be instructed on proper administration and side effects, including the following instructions.

- Take prednisone with food or milk to lessen stomach upset.
- Swallow prednisone tablets with a full glass of water.
- Let your doctor or nurse know about all medications you are taking before starting prednisone and any new medications that may be prescribed by another healthcare provider while you are taking prednisone.
- Do not stop taking prednisone suddenly. You may need a gradual reduction in dosage before you stop completely. Contact your doctor or nurse for instructions.

Long-term use of prednisone may result in side effects. Patients should be advised about the following side effects of prednisone therapy.

- Prednisone weakens the body's immune system and may reduce your body's ability to fight infection. Contact your doctor or nurse immediately if you have signs of infection (fever over 100.5°F [38°C], cough, pain or burning on urination, diarrhea, or signs of an infection in a cut or wound).
- Do not receive immunizations while taking prednisone without talking with your doctor or nurse first.
- If you experience any of the following serious side effects, stop taking prednisone and contact your doctor or nurse immediately:

  - Hives, difficulty breathing, closing of your throat, swelling of lips, tongue, or face
  - Increase in your blood pressure, severe headache, or blurred vision
  - Sudden weight gain (more than five pounds in one to two days).

Prednisone has other less serious side effects that are more likely to occur, such as
- Insomnia (difficulty sleeping)
- Nausea, vomiting, or dyspepsia (stomach upset, indigestion)
- Fatigue
- Muscle weakness or joint pain
- Increased hunger or thirst
- Hyperglycemia (high blood sugar).
  Less frequent side effects include
- Acne
- Increased hair growth
- Thinning of the skin
- Osteoporosis
- Cushingoid appearance (round face, humpback)
- Changes in behavior.

A printable patient teaching sheet from Sanofi-Aventis with instructions on taking dexamethasone during docetaxel therapy can be accessed online (http://taxotere.com/docs/pdf/prostate.pdf).

Hyperglycemia is a known adverse side effect of prednisone and dexamethasone and may also exacerbate latent diabetes mellitus (impaired glucose tolerance). Nurses caring for diabetic patients on a regimen that includes a corticosteroid should pay special attention to patient education concerning diabetes management (Kuck, 2006; Pandit, Burke, Gustafson, Minocha, & Peiris, 1993). Corticosteroids can cause transient hyperglycemia, and patients who have managed their diabetes by lifestyle methods (i.e., diet and exercise) may need to add an oral antihyperglycemic or injectable insulin in order to ensure adequate glycemic control. Advising the patient's primary healthcare provider of the prednisone therapy, including the dose and duration, will help in multidisciplinary management of the patient's diabetes. Regular monitoring of blood glucose levels in the clinic setting is advisable (Campbell & Braithwaite, 2004; Gallagher & Gapstur, 2006; Mathis & Liu, 2005).

Radiation

External beam radiation therapy (EBRT) and brachytherapy are options for management of clinically localized and metastatic prostate cancer. Significant changes in treatment approach have taken place in the past 10 years, yet no clear consensus exists as to the best RT option. Treatment decisions should be made based on individual patient needs, prior treatment, and the patient's condition.

Assessment

Pre-RT assessment should include a complete physical examination, including assessment of the abdomen, rectum, scrotum, and perineal area, to identify any abnormalities that would interfere with treatment or recovery following the procedure. Patient history of illnesses and surgeries and a complete, current medication list should be obtained. A baseline assessment of urinary symptoms is important, as it may be indicative of the degree of urinary morbidity following treatment with RT. It may be helpful to determine a patient's American Urological Association (AUA) score upon initial evaluation and during follow-up exams after intervention. Consisting of seven questions, the current AUA scoring system attempts to gauge the extent to which one is experiencing urinary difficulty by scoring each response in the form of a numeric value (Nitti, Kim, & Combs, 1994). Originally derived from a more extensive survey to determine the degree of bothersome urinary symptoms experienced by patients with benign prostatic hypertrophy, the AUA index has demonstrated high internal consistency (Cronbach's alpha = 0.86) and high test-retest reliability (r = .92) (Barry et al., 1992). It is believed that patients with a higher pretreatment AUA score may have a higher degree of urinary morbidity secondary to RT or other interventions.

Depending on the severity of symptoms, patients with irritable bowel disease, active diverticulitis, and ulcerative colitis may not be candidates for EBRT or brachytherapy. In addition, patients with a history of TURP may be excluded from treatment with brachytherapy. Ultimately, the resulting glandular deficit following TURP should be determined by transrectal ultrasound before proceeding with interstitial prostate brachytherapy. In some cases, interstitial implants can be given despite history of TURP, especially if the TURP was performed in the distant past. A systems review with a careful exploration of urinary and sexual function to document baseline function is needed. Social history of smoking or alcohol consumption should be assessed.

Radiation Safety

Patients undergoing EBRT do not require any instructions regarding radiation safety. The dose and method of administration do not result in high levels of radioactivity in the patient. Specific guidelines are available for patients undergoing permanent radioactive seed implants (brachytherapy) (see Figure 5-1). Healthcare providers must follow the institutional guidelines at their place of employment to ensure personal safety. Guidelines for healthcare provider safety when caring for patients undergoing brachytherapy are found in Figure 5-2.

Symptom Management

Adverse effects of RT vary according to the treatment method employed but may include diarrhea, nausea and

---

Figure 5-1. Radiation Safety Instructions for Patients Following Prostate Brachytherapy

Most patients undergoing prostate brachytherapy are discharged home as soon as they are stable following the procedure. It is important to educate patients and family members about radiation safety for the recommended period of 8 weeks following the procedure. The following rules for post-implant in-home safety follow the radiation exposure principles of *as low as reasonably achievable* (ALARA) and should be provided to patients.

For 8 weeks following your seed implant procedure:
- Maintain a distance of at least 4–6 feet from others. If this distance is maintained, contact is permissible for an unlimited amount of time.
- Strive for quick hellos, hugs, and kisses; avoid prolonged close contact with anyone.
- Infants, children, and pregnant women should not sit on your lap or lay up against you.
- Sleeping alone is recommended.
- Wear a condom during sexual intercourse, once the radiation oncologist advises that sexual intercourse is safe, as seeds may pass from the body in semen.
- No special precautions are needed for body fluids (urine, feces, semen, blood, saliva, or sweat). They are not radioactive. Double flushing is not required. You may be asked to strain your urine for the first 1–2 weeks following the procedure to watch for seeds that pass in the urine.
- If seeds pass in the urine during voiding, do not pick up or touch the seed with your hands. Use tweezers to place the seed in the receptacle provided and return it to the radiation oncology department for disposal. Do not flush the seed down the toilet.
- Seeds are made of thin silver metal and resemble thin wires, similar in size and shape to a grain of rice. They will not activate airport or security metal detectors.

Note. Based on information from Cattani et al., 2006; Lee & Frank, 2006; Speight & Roach, 2005.

---

vomiting, fatigue, proctitis, cystitis, urinary dysfunction, ED, or skin reactions. Nurses in urology, medical oncology, and RT share the responsibility of educating patients with prostate cancer on safety and management of RT-related side effects. A multidisciplinary approach to patient management will achieve more positive outcomes for the patients.

Patient education should include the specific treatment modality, goal of therapy, length of treatment in terms of each session and overall regimen, and the anticipated side effects of EBRT (see Table 5-4) and brachytherapy (see Table 5-5). Explaining the various equipment and activities of personnel in the area of the treatment room will help to relieve patients' concerns when treatment actually begins (Iwamoto & Maher, 2001). Fatigue is a common side effect of RT, and many patients express concern that their nutritional intake may be the cause of fatigue and ask about vitamins or nutritional supplements. A double-blind, randomized crossover

---

Figure 5-2. Instructions for Healthcare Providers Caring for Prostate Brachytherapy Patients

1. Put on protective gloves before entering the patient's room. Although passage of a brachytherapy seed in urine is unlikely, absorption of radioactivity is easily prevented by wearing gloves.
2. Work quickly, but effectively and courteously. Minimize your time in the room.
3. Maintain the greatest distance possible from the patient consistent with effective care. Radiation exposure drops off drastically with increasing distance.
4. Controversy exists regarding exposure of pregnant or lactating staff to implant patients. Anterior skin surface exposure rates suggest that exposure to the general public is not a significant concern. Healthcare occupational exposure risk is considered low, and individual institutional policy, based on the half-life of the radiation source used, usually dictates staff exposure precautions. Studies to determine exposure rates to pregnant and lactating staff during or shortly after prostate brachytherapy are lacking.
5. Make use of portable lead shielding whenever possible.
6. Leave all trash, linens, and food trays in the room. Upon leaving the room, remove gloves and place them in the trash receptacles inside the room. Radiation safety should survey all materials before they leave the room.
7. After leaving the room, wash your hands.
8. In the event a seed becomes dislodged, notify radiation therapy *immediately*. Do not permit others to enter the room until the seed is secured. Do not attempt to handle a dislodged implant or applicator unless you are specially trained to do so.

Note. Based on information from Cattani et al., 2006; Michalski et al., 2003; Smathers et al., 1999.

---

trial of multivitamin versus placebo in patients with breast cancer undergoing RT reported that multivitamin intake did not improve RT-related fatigue (de Souza Fede et al., 2007). Limitations of this study that may affect generalization to prostate cancer are small size (N = 40) and study population (breast cancer).

Brachytherapy Considerations

Patient teaching for brachytherapy should take place before the procedure and should be reinforced with verbal and written instructions prior to discharge. Goals during the period following the procedure include pain management and return to normal function as quickly as possible. A post-implant computed tomography scan is obtained to verify the seed placement, and the urinary catheter is removed thereafter. The patient must urinate before being discharged to ensure there is no urinary retention. Patients should be instructed to drink at least one to two liters of fluid daily for two to three days following discharge, if cardiac capacity allows. The urologist or APN will prescribe an antibiotic. Patients generally are discharged on acetaminophen or an NSAID with instructions to contact the nurse or physician if pain is not controlled after

returning home. The procedural discomfort usually resolves within a few days (Behrend, 2005). Additional discharge instructions should include notifying the physician or nurse if any of the following occur:
- Difficulty urinating or blood in the urine
- Chest pain, cough, or shortness of breath
- Nausea or vomiting
- Unusual bleeding or bruises
- Fever above 101°F (38°C)

As part of postbrachytherapy assessment, inspection of the perineal area may reveal tenderness, ecchymosis, or edema below the scrotum. Some men may experience hematuria following removal of the indwelling catheter and during the first 24–48 hours at home, and a small percentage may experience rectal irritation or bleeding. Dysuria and frequency of urination may be present beginning 10–14 days after implantation and gradually decreases as the radiation dose emitted by the seeds decreases over time. Edema may be more severe at night, thus increasing nighttime urinary symptoms (Lee & Frank, 2006; Loeb & Nadler, 2006).

Radiopharmaceuticals

Three radiopharmaceutical agents currently are FDA-approved for the treatment of metastatic bone pain: phosphorus-32 (^{32}P), strontium-89 (^{89}Sr), and samarium-153 (^{153}Sm- ethylene diamine tetramethylene phosphonate [^{153}Sm-EDTMP]). These agents localize to regions of enhanced bone turnover and deliver high local doses of radiation through the emission of beta particles, causing destruction and shrinkage of cancer cells, resulting in pain relief. Treatment is palliative, not curative, and is an accepted method for palliation of painful bone metastases in patients with metastatic prostate cancer. These agents generally are well tolerated but cause hematologic toxicity, primarily thrombocytopenia, because of the radiation effects on bone marrow. Toxicity for ^{153}Sm appears to be less than that for ^{89}Sr because of the shorter half-life and shorter range of emitted energy in ^{153}Sm (Berthold et al., 2005). Repeat doses of ^{153}Sm can safely be given, provided that white blood cell and platelet counts are normal prior to administration (Sartor, Reid, Higano, Bushnell, & Quick, 2005).

Liepe, Runge, and Kotzerke (2005) evaluated the safety and efficacy of rhenium-188 hydroxyethylidene diphosphonate, rhenium-186 hydroxyethylidene diphosphonate, and ^{89}Sr on pain symptoms, QOL, and bone marrow function in patients with breast and prostate cancer. Pain relief ranged from 67%–77% among the three agents. No significant differences occurred in bone marrow toxicity; the maximum platelet and leukocyte nadirs were observed between the second and fifth weeks after treatment and were reversible within 12 weeks (Liepe et al.). A clinical trial of ^{153}Sm combined with docetaxel in patients with HRPC demonstrated that ^{153}Sm, if adequately combined with chemotherapy, had some clinical benefit in terms of regression and prolonged survival. Toxici-

Table 5-4. Management of Acute Side Effects of External Beam Radiation Therapy		
Body System	**Symptom**	**Nursing Interventions**
Gastrointestinal	Diarrhea	Assess baseline stool pattern; define diarrhea for patient; assess current stool pattern throughout radiation therapy (RT). Assess perianal skin irritation. Have patient consume low-residue diet. Maintain hydration with 1–2 liters fluid daily. Administer antidiarrheal medication PRN: loperamide; diphenoxylate plus atropine; consider octreotide if refractory. Add psyllium fiber to antidiarrheal therapy to encourage formed stool.
	Proctitis	Assess for rectal discomfort or history of hemorrhoids. Assess perianal skin irritation. Consult with RT personnel for approved topical skin preparations; use PRN after RT treatment. Give tepid sitz baths QID PRN. Consider topical steroid cream or suppository (hydrocortisone 2.5%) if approved by radiation oncologist or radiation nurse.
Genitourinary	Cystitis	Assess baseline urinary frequency, nocturia, incontinence, and dysuria. Collect urine specimen to assess for urinary tract infection (UTI). Maintain hydration with 1–2 liters fluid daily. Consider nonsteroidal anti-inflammatory drugs (NSAIDs) or bladder analgesics unless contraindicated.
	Urinary dysfunction Frequent urination Nocturia Incontinence Dysuria	Assess baseline urinary frequency, nocturia, incontinence, and dysuria. Collect urine specimen to assess for UTI. Maintain hydration with 1–2 liters fluid daily. Consider NSAIDs or bladder analgesics unless contraindicated. For nocturia or urinary frequency caused by incomplete emptying of bladder, consider alpha-1 blockers (terazosin, doxazosin) or alpha-1A blocker (tamsulosin). Consider condom catheter or incontinence pads/garments; bladder training.
	Erectile dysfunction (ED)	Assess baseline erectile function and current concerns. Openly discuss issues and concerns with patient and partner. Consider referral to urologist or ED specialist to discuss management and treatment options.
Dermatologic	Skin reaction	Assess gluteal skinfold at baseline and at regular intervals throughout RT. Give tepid sitz baths QID PRN. Consult with RT personnel for approved topical skin preparations; use PRN after RT treatment.
Constitutional	Fatigue	Assess baseline level of activity, energy, and fatigue. Evaluate comorbid conditions that may induce fatigue. Evaluate concomitant medications that may induce fatigue. Maintain adequate, high-quality nutritional intake. Maintain hydration. Recommend energy-conserving measures: regular, moderate exercise, adequate rest and sleep, stress reduction.

Note. Based on information from Boehmer et al., 2006; Held-Warmkessel, 2005; Incrocci, 2006; Iwamoto & Maher, 2001; Lee & Frank, 2006; Loeb & Nadler, 2006; Su & Jani, 2007.

ties of the combination regimen were mild and comparable to those observed when the two therapies were used separately (Mariani et al., 2006). An alpha-emitting investigational agent, radium-223, has shown promising phase II results with little or no myelotoxic effect (Nilsson et al., 2007).

Assessment

The dominant site of metastases in men with prostate cancer is the bone. Because of the lack of other measur-able disease, response parameters for prostate cancer differ from those for other solid tumors. Response to treatment of HRPC bone metastases is assessed by palliative end points: decreased pain, improved QOL, and potentially prolonged survival. Therefore, pain assessment as a measure of response to therapy and evaluation of patient QOL is quite important. Assessment of baseline pain as a presenting symptom or as a surrogate marker for progression and follow-up assessments at predetermined intervals are requisite components of oncology

Table 5-5. Management of Acute Side Effects of Prostate Brachytherapy

Body System	Symptom	Nursing Interventions
Constitutional	Fatigue	Assess baseline level of activity, energy, and fatigue. Evaluate comorbid conditions that may induce fatigue. Evaluate concomitant medications that may induce fatigue. Maintain adequate, high-quality nutritional intake. Maintain hydration. Recommend energy-conserving measures: pacing activities and regular, moderate exercise after recovery from implant procedure; adequate rest and sleep; stress reduction.
	Pain, perineal	Assess baseline pain prior to brachytherapy; assess patient prior pain management and pain tolerance; educate patient on 0–10 pain scale. Intermittent ice pack to perineum for first 24 hours after the procedure. Administer pain medication as ordered.
Genitourinary	Cystitis	Assess baseline urinary frequency, nocturia, incontinence, and dysuria. Collect urine specimen to assess for urinary tract infection (UTI). Maintain hydration with 1–2 liters fluid daily. Consider nonsteroidal anti-inflammatory drugs (NSAIDs) or bladder analgesics unless contraindicated.
	Urinary dysfunction • Frequent urination • Nocturia • Incontinence • Dysuria	Assess baseline urinary frequency, nocturia, incontinence, and dysuria. Collect urine specimen to assess for UTI. Maintain hydration with 1–2 liters fluid daily. Consider NSAIDs or bladder analgesics unless contraindicated. For nocturia or urinary frequency caused by incomplete emptying of bladder, consider alpha-1 blockers (terazosin, doxazosin) or alpha-1A blocker (tamsulosin). Consider condom catheter or incontinence pads/garments; bladder training.
	Hematuria	Maintain hydration with 1–2 liters fluid daily. Instruct patient to contact doctor or nurse immediately if unable to void or experiencing significant pelvic or bladder pain. Collect urine specimen to assess for UTI. Continuous bladder irrigation until urine clears (inpatient only). Instruct patient to avoid strenuous activity and heavy lifting for 2–3 days following procedure.
	Urinary retention	Make certain that patient can void freely before leaving procedure area (voiding trial). If unable to void, insert indwelling catheter for 24–48 hours and repeat voiding trial. If unsuccessful, instruct patient on intermittent catheterization and assist patient to obtain supplies. Record time and amount of voids. Suprapubic catheter is indicated if patient cannot perform self-catheterization.
	Erectile dysfunction (ED)	Assess baseline erectile function and current concerns. Openly discuss issues and concerns with patient and partner. Consider referral to urologist or ED specialist to discuss management and treatment options.
Gastrointestinal	Proctitis Constipation Diarrhea	Assess for rectal discomfort or history of hemorrhoids. Assess perianal skin irritation. Avoid constipation with use of stool softener, increased dietary fiber, and hydration. Have patient consume low-residue diet if ≥ 4 stools per day. Administer antidiarrheal medication PRN. Consider topical steroid cream or suppository (hydrocortisone 2.5%) if approved by radiation oncologist or radiation nurse. Give tepid sitz baths QID PRN.

Note. Based on information from Lee & Frank, 2006; Loeb & Nadler, 2006; Speight & Roach, 2005; Stipetich et al., 2002.

nursing assessment. Sequential documentation of pain assessments in the medical record will facilitate multidisciplinary care of patients with HRPC.

Any patient with advanced prostate cancer reporting new-onset back pain, numbness or tingling in the arms or legs, or change in urinary or bowel function must immediately be evaluated for spinal cord compression (SCC). SCC is an oncologic emergency, and delay in diagnosis and treatment can result in permanent neurologic damage and loss of function. Diagnosis of SCC is made by magnetic resonance imaging or myelogram. Treatment for SCC includes dexamethasone to decrease edema, RT, external bracing, and pain management. In some cases, surgery may be used. Nursing management should focus on changes in neurologic functioning, preserving function, restoring lost function, and assisting in adaptation to changes in function (Held-Warmkessel, 2005).

Side Effect Management

Evaluation of side effects to radionuclide administration is essential. Before radionuclide therapy is administered, consideration should be given to the patient's current clinical and hematologic status and bone marrow response to prior treatment with myelotoxic agents. Metastatic prostate cancer can be associated with disseminated intravascular coagulation (DIC); caution should be exercised in treating patients whose platelet counts are falling or who have other clinical or laboratory findings suggesting DIC. Because of the unknown potential for additive effects on bone marrow, radionuclides should not be given concurrently with chemotherapy or EBRT unless the clinical benefits outweigh the risks (Amersham Healthcare, 1998; Berthold et al., 2005; Cytogen Corp., 2003). Myelosuppression is a known side effect of beta-emitting therapies. A CBC with differential and platelet count should be obtained as a baseline before the administration of a radiopharmaceutical and weekly for at least eight weeks or until recovery of adequate bone marrow function is evident (Cytogen Corp.). A flushing sensation has been observed in patients following a rapid (less than 30-second injection) administration (Amersham Healthcare).

Radiation Safety

Special precautions, such as urinary catheterization, should be taken following radionuclide administration to patients who are incontinent to minimize the risk of radioactive contamination of clothing, bed linen, and the patient's environment (Amersham Healthcare, 1998). Patients being discharged following the administration of radiopharmaceuticals and their family members should be educated on radiation safety procedures (see Figure 5-3). Safety data information for ^{89}Sr (Amersham Healthcare) and ^{153}Sm-EDTMP (Cytogen Corp., 2003) are available online through the respective pharmaceutical company Web sites or from the RT or nuclear medicine department in the treatment facility. A safety data sheet for ^{32}P is available through the manufacturer, PerkinElmer, Inc. (2007).

Figure 5-3. Patient and Family Instructions Following Radiopharmaceutical Administration

The medication given to relieve your bone pain contains a small amount of radioactivity that is eliminated from your body in your urine over the next 7–10 days. You will need to follow these precautions to keep yourself and your family members or caregivers safe.

- Flush the toilet twice after voiding or having a bowel movement.
- Make sure you wash your hands well after using the bathroom.
- Do not use a urinal.
- If you find that you are incontinent, contact your doctor or nurse for recommendation for a special type of catheter that can be used at home.
- If you are incontinent, clean up spilled urine from the floor or surfaces immediately and discard the paper towels or cloths in a plastic bag. The bag may be discarded in your ordinary trash.
- If bed linens or clothing become soiled with urine or blood, wash them separately from general laundry.
- The medication will affect how well your bone marrow makes blood cells, putting you at increased risk for infection, bleeding, and fatigue. The effect on your bone marrow is temporary and will be monitored by your doctor or nurse through regular blood tests. Contact your doctor or nurse immediately if you develop a fever, chills, or other signs of infection, bleeding, or extreme fatigue.

Note. Based on information from Amersham Healthcare, 1998; Cytogen Corp., 2003; Iwamoto & Maher, 2001.

Common Treatment-Related Morbidities

Genitourinary Side Effects of Treatment

As previously discussed, regardless of which intervention is decided upon, nearly all men receiving treatment for prostate cancer will experience some degree of urinary morbidity and sexual dysfunction.

Assessment of Genitourinary Function

Because urinary incontinence and problems of sexual functioning (sexual desire, orgasm, and ability to achieve and maintain an erection) are reported side effects of most prostate cancer treatment modalities, the oncology nurse must assess pretreatment function to establish a baseline against which to evaluate posttreatment function. The physical examination should include examination of the abdomen and genitalia and assessment of peripheral pulses and blood pressure. Laboratory tests to rule out systemic diseases, such as diabetes and thyroid abnormalities, and a complete listing of concomitant medications are necessary to rule out secondary causes of ED.

Sexuality is a complex phenomenon encompassing identity, body image, relationships, sexual activity, and communication (Katz, 2005). Men and their partners may be embarrassed and reluctant to bring up topics of sexuality and incontinence with care providers and may assume that little can be done to alleviate these problems. Survival concerns combined with potential embarrassment associated with discussions of sexual activity, especially among older couples, may keep patients from asking questions about incontinence and ED or may prevent them from fully understanding the information that is supplied. Before beginning discussions with the patient and partner, nurses need to assess how much partner involvement is desired. They need to ask targeted questions about the importance of sexual activity for both the patient and the partner before beginning patient education (Docherty, Brothwell, & Symons, 2007). The PLISSIT model for sexual assessment and intervention (Annon, 1976) is a method to gather assessment data and provide related interventions. Using this model allows for a more comfortable engagement between the clinician and patient by giving permission to the individual or couple to ask questions and discuss sexuality (see Figure 5-4). Giving permission to talk about sexual and other sensitive, private issues might be handled by making a statement as follows: "Many men (couples) have questions about prostate cancer and sexual activity. Do you have any questions or concerns?" The nurse is giving the patient or couple permission to discuss a topic that they may consider embarrassing, and they, in turn, give permission to the nurse to discuss these topics by virtue of their questions. Johnson (2004) suggested the following interview approach: (1) provide privacy, (2) promote a comfortable atmosphere, and (3) ask clear and direct questions. She also suggested that the nurse remind individuals that they do not have to answer any specific question. The oncology nurse may participate in the assessment steps of PLISSIT and refer the patient and partner to ongoing counseling with a qualified sex counselor or therapist. A listing of professional resources can be found on the Web site for the American Association of Sexuality Educators, Counselors, and Therapists (www.aasect.org). Tiefer and Schuetz-Mueller (1995) suggested a series of direct and nonjudgmental sexual history questions to discuss with men with prostate cancer who are experiencing ED (see Figure 5-5). For couples who are not interested in pharmacologic or mechanical solutions to ED, counseling with an emphasis on communication skills and sensate focus exercises is helpful

---

Figure 5-5. Sexual History for Men With Prostate Cancer and Erectile Dysfunction

1. Describe what happens when you try to have sex.
2. Is your penis firm enough to go inside your partner?
3. Is your penis firm when you awaken in the morning or during masturbation?
4. Can you have an orgasm?
5. How long have you had difficulty getting and keeping an erection?
6. Did you have problems with erections before your prostate cancer treatment?
7. What do you think is causing your difficulty in getting and keeping an erection?
8. How has this affected you and your partner?
9. How has this affected your relationship with your partner?
10. Have you tried any treatments? If so, what, and did you have any success?

Note. Based on information from Tiefer & Schuetz-Mueller, 1995.

---

in finding alternatives to sexual intercourse and maintaining intimacy (Katz, 2005). Older men may have experienced incontinence and ED prior to treatment and may assume that worsening symptoms are the result of age, not treatment. Some men may not complain, adopting an attitude of survival at any cost and accepting any and all side effects without complaint. The opinion and observations of the patient's partner also are important for an accurate assessment (Katz, 2007b).

Rosen, Althof, and Giuliano (2006) published a summary of the most commonly used self-report instruments for the diagnosis of ED and assessment of treatment efficacy. Patient event logs and diaries are valuable research tools for the collection of specific information about individual sexual experiences, as they do not rely on patient memories across extensive periods and record data related to a key treatment outcome for ED, namely, successful sexual intercourse attempts (Rosen et al., 2006). Examples of validated assessment tools to establish baseline and continuing sexual and urinary function include

- The National Survey of Prostate Disease and Quality of Life (NCI, 2007b)
- The Prostate Cancer Index (Litwin, 2002).

Using an assessment tool to evaluate erectile function over time and throughout treatment may be helpful. The abridged International Index of Erectile Function (IIEF), the IIEF-5 (Rosen, Cappelleri, Smith, Lipsky, & Pena, 1999) (see Figure 5-6), is easily administered in the office setting and rates a total of five questions on a Likert scale: the lower the score, the more significant the degree of ED.

Interventions for Urinary Incontinence

Urinary incontinence is a common side effect following prostatectomy, cryosurgery, or RT. Stress incontinence is the most common type of incontinence after prostate surgery, although some patients also report mixed incontinence

---

Figure 5-4. The PLISSIT Model for Sexual Assessment and Intervention

Permission to ask and to give information
Limited **I**nformation about sexual concerns or questions
Giving **S**pecific **S**uggestions in response to questions about sexuality
Providing **I**ntensive **T**herapy for sexual issues of the individual or couple

Note. Based on information from Annon, 1976.

Figure 5-6. International Index of Erectile Function-5 (IIEF-5)				
The IIEF-5 score is the sum of the ordinal responses (**bold**) to the items below. The score can range from 5 to 25. Erectile dysfunction is classified into five severity levels, ranging from none (22–25) through severe (5–7). **Over the past four weeks:**				
How do you rate your confidence that you could get and keep an erection?	Very low **1**	Low **2**	Moderate **3**	High **4**	Very high **5**
When you had erections with sexual stimulation, how often were your erections hard enough for penetration (hard enough to enter your partner)?	Almost never/ never **1**	A few times (much less than half the time) **2**	Sometimes (about half the time) **3**	Most times (much more than half the time) **4**	Almost always/ always **5**
During sexual intercourse, how often were you able to maintain your erection after you had penetrated (entered) your partner?	Almost never/ never **1**	A few times (much less than half the time) **2**	Sometimes (about half the time) **3**	Most times (much more than half the time) **4**	Almost always/ always **5**
During sexual intercourse, how difficult was it to maintain your erection to completion of intercourse?	Extremely difficult **1**	Very difficult **2**	Difficult **3**	Slightly difficult **4**	Not difficult **5**
When you attempted sexual intercourse, how often was it satisfactory for you?	Almost never/ never **1**	A few times (much less than half the time) **2**	Sometimes (about half the time) **3**	Most times (much more than half the time) **4**	Almost always/ always **5**
Note. From "Development and Evaluation of an Abridged, 5-Item Version of the International Index of Erectile Function (IIEF-5) as a Diagnostic Tool for Erectile Dysfunction," by R.C. Rosen, J.C. Cappelleri, M.D. Smith, J. Lipsky, and B.M. Pena, 1999, *International Journal of Impotence Research, 11*(6), p. 322. Copyright 1999 by Macmillan Publishers Ltd. Adapted with permission.				

(Palmer, Fogarty, Somerfield, & Powel, 2003) (see Table 5-6). The least invasive techniques for management of urinary incontinence are wearing a continence pad, diaper, or condom catheter to contain urine. For many men, these are not acceptable. Other options include conservative measures such as Kegel exercises, biofeedback, and medications. Scheduled toileting involves a regular voiding regimen and typically is recommended for frail individuals and older adults. Bladder retraining uses scheduled toileting but gradually extends urination to longer intervals. Toileting techniques are effective in treating urge and mixed incontinence but seldom are effective in stress incontinence following prostatectomy. Depending on symptoms, medications can help men with incontinence. Anticholinergic agents can be used as first-line treatments for urge incontinence because they inhibit detrusor contraction and may help to increase bladder capacity, but they are less effective in stress incontinence. Biofeedback can help men to gain awareness and control of their urinary tract muscles. The principle of biofeedback is simple: A variety of instruments are used to record small electrical signals that are emitted when specific muscles are contracted to urinate. These muscle contractions then are converted into audio or visual signals

that patients can recognize and learn in order to control muscular activity. Palmer et al., in a survey regarding management strategies used for urinary incontinence occurring after prostatectomy, found that 54% of subjects self-reported using behavioral strategies such as Kegel exercises, although usage appeared to decline over time. Sitting to void, which may empty the bladder more effectively, was a method used by all groups, and its usage appeared to increase over time from surgery. More than half of the men used containment strategies, such as pads.

Stress incontinence typically is treated with surgery. Accepted surgical options include bulking agents, such as collagen. Urethral compression through placement of a fixed compression device, such as an artificial urinary sphincter, is the primary surgical intervention for urinary incontinence following prostatectomy (Castle et al., 2005). Fixed compressive devices confer continence by obstructing outflow, but this resistance often is overcome when sufficient elevation of intra-abdominal pressure occurs (e.g., sneezing, coughing, lifting heavy objects). Dynamic compressive devices use variations in pressure that can be modified to achieve continence. The classic dynamic device is the AMS-800® (American Medical

Table 5-6. Types of Urinary Incontinence		
Type of Incontinence	**Symptoms**	**Cause**
Stress incontinence	Urine leakage when patient coughs, laughs, sneezes, or exercises	Muscle or nerve damage to urinary sphincter
Overflow incontinence	Difficulty starting urine stream
Dribbling stream with little force	Blockage or stricture of urethra because of tumor blockage or scar tissue
Urge incontinence	Sudden need to urinate	Sensitivity of bladder to stretching as bladder becomes full
Note. Based on information from McGuire, 2005; Palmer et al., 2003.		

Systems) artificial urinary sphincter. Castle et al. reported on perineal bone anchor slings in males with postprostatectomy incontinence, noting that the procedure was most successful in mild to moderate incontinence, success declined with time, and problems with bone and perineal pain developed after the procedure.

In summary, the overall effectiveness of conservative management of urinary incontinence following prostatectomy remains unclear, and further phase III trials are needed to fully evaluate current interventions (Hunter, Moore, & Glazener, 2007). Stress incontinence, the most common type of incontinence after prostatectomy, typically is treated with surgery. Severe incontinence may require urinary diversion (ileal conduit) (Ahmed & Davies, 2005). Patients with persistent incontinence should be referred to a WOC nurse for consultation.

Sexual Dysfunction

Sexual functions include desire (libido), orgasm, and the ability to have an erection (Katz, 2007a). ADT has a global effect on sexual functioning. Dahn et al. (2004) examined the relationship between libido and ED and found that men with low or no libido have less distress when they experience ED than men who still desire sex but have ED. Additionally, men with lower levels of sexual functioning had significantly lower QOL scores as the level of sexual desire increased, suggesting that desire in the absence of adequate functioning may result in poorer QOL. Men with better sexual functioning tended to have higher QOL scores as the level of sexual desire increased (Dahn et al.).

Excessive RT to the proximal penis has been implicated in brachytherapy-related ED. RT-related ED generally is thought to be caused by chronic hypoxia in the corporal smooth muscle of the penis with a subsequent loss of elasticity and distensibility, which could lead to venous leak (Stipetich et al., 2005). Postoperative fibrosis also is believed to cause penile shortening, observed in 68% of men three months after nerve-sparing radical retropubic prostatectomy (Savoie, Kim, & Soloway, 2003). The oncology nurse, in conjunction with the physician, should encourage patients to attain regular

erections with or without sexual relations (Merrick, Butler, & Wallner, 2005). The absence of routine penile erections is thought to contribute to chronic hypoxia of the corporal smooth muscle and venous leak (Savoie et al.). Based on the premise that erections enhance tissue oxygenation and suppress smooth muscle fibrosis, nocturnal erections may have therapeutic benefit. In a phase III placebo-controlled clinical trial, Montorsi et al. (2000) demonstrated that sildenafil taken at bedtime produced a significant improvement in nocturnal erectile activity over placebo. Sildenafil in men with ED following RT (EBRT or brachytherapy) was shown to improve erectile function, with the best efficacy demonstrated earlier in the 36-month follow-up period in the study (Ohebshalom, Parker, Guhring, & Mulhall, 2005).

Following prostatectomy, orgasm is still possible despite lack of erections, but men will no longer experience ejaculation because of the removal of the seminal vesicles (Hollenbeck, Dunn, Wei, Montie, & Sanda, 2003). It is important to provide patients with this information as part of the informed consent process prior to surgery because most men will assume that they will no longer experience orgasm if they have ED. Although orgasmic function may be preserved, a qualitative change may occur in the experience of orgasm, with the man experiencing less propulsive sensation and possible pelvic pain of variable duration (Katz, 2007b). The recovery of sexual function following prostatectomy depends on a variety of factors, such as the following (Hollenbeck et al.; Madsen & Ganey-Code, 2006; Stanford et al., 2000).

- Age (younger men have more success)
- Preoperative sexual functioning
- Smaller prostate gland resections (smaller size prostate gland resections have better outcomes)
- Surgical technique (nerve-sparing procedures have better outcomes)

Sexual dysfunction can persist for years following surgery, with the greatest recovery occurring in the first five years (Penson et al., 2005). Bokhour, Clark, Inui, Silliman, and Talcott (2001) reported negative changes in social and intimate relationships and alteration in masculine self-concept.

Interventions for Sexual Dysfunction

The most difficult side effect of ADT to treat is loss of libido, which occurs in approximately 54% of men treated with ADT monotherapy (Potosky et al., 2002); 5%–30% treated with antiandrogen monotherapy (See et al., 2002); and 90% of men treated with combined GnRH agonist/antiandrogen therapy (See et al.; Wirth et al., 2005). Loss of libido differs from ED, which is the inability to achieve an erection. Erections can be achieved in the absence of libido; however, many men lose interest in sexual activity when libido is absent. No effective medical therapy exists for altered libido in the setting of prostate cancer. Libido is dependent on adequate levels of testosterone. The goal of ADT therapy is to decrease testosterone levels in order to cut off the hormone supply to prostate cancer cells; therefore, treating altered libido with supplemental testosterone is not an option. Intermittent ADT has been shown to improve or restore potency during the off-therapy periods (Bruchovsky et al., 2007; Tunn, 2007). Psychosocial counseling may help; referral to a sex counselor or therapist would be appropriate for couples willing to undergo sex therapy.

Treatment of ED focuses on two primary modalities: pharmacologic and mechanical assistive devices and procedures. Phosphodiesterase-5 inhibitor (PDE5-I) medications act by causing relaxation of smooth muscle in the corpus cavernosa of the penis, allowing blood to enter the spongy tissue during sexual stimulation. Although three PDE5-I medications (see Table 5-7) currently are available in the United States, no direct comparisons have been performed in men following radical prostatectomy. Response is dependent on the type of surgery, patient age, and preoperative erectile functioning (Raina et al., 2004). Specific contraindications for the use of PDE5-I therapy include thromboembolic events such as stroke; MI; recent significant cardiac arrhythmias; persistent hypo- or hypertension; cardiac failure; and patients on concomitant nitrates or alpha-blockers (Shabsigh, 2004; Weeks & Ficorelli, 2006a). Patients prefer oral medications over mechanical methods of ED treatment because they are easy to use and noninvasive and allow for spontaneity (Katz, 2007b). Mechanical devices (see Table 5-8) include vacuum constriction pumps, intraurethral prostaglandin, intracavernosal injections of alprostadil, or penile implants. Oncology nurses counseling men with ED should consider oral PDE5-I therapy first and then progress through a treatment plan utilizing more invasive methods if PDE5-I therapy is ineffective or contraindicated (Katz, 2007b).

Important to remember is that urinary continence and sexual functioning are seen as essential constructs of adulthood and masculinity, and loss of these functions is seen as a threat to manhood (McGuire, 2005; Palmer et al., 2003; Paterson, 2000; Stanford et al., 2000). Specific education for oncology nurses in areas of male sexual function, specializing in the unique difficulties that men face while undergoing treatment for prostate cancer, would benefit these men and their partners throughout the continuum of care from diagnosis to decision making to long-term care (Navon & Morag, 2003). Oncology nursing interventions that focus on provision of relevant information and counseling can positively affect patient and partner health-related QOL.

Cancer Therapy–Induced Bone Loss

Long-term use of ADT is associated with a decrease in bone mineral density (BMD), resulting in osteopenia or osteoporosis (Guise, 2006; Shahinian et al., 2005). Androgens mediate osteoblast proliferation and bone development; ADT causes a 3%–5% annual BMD decrease (Ross & Small, 2002). Shahinian et al. conducted a retrospective chart review of men (N = 50,613) treated with ADT for prostate cancer, finding that 19.4% of men who received ADT had at least one fracture, compared with 12.6% of men who did not receive ADT (p < .001). The relative risk of any fracture or a fracture that resulted in hospitalization increased steadily with the increasing number of doses of GnRH agonist received during the first year after diagnosis. The relative risk of any fracture was 1.45 (95% CI = 1.36–1.56) among those receiving nine or more doses of GnRH agonist in the first 12 months after diagnosis, and 1.54 (95% CI = 1.42–1.68) among those who underwent orchiectomy (Shahinian et al.). Men who show evidence of osteopenia or osteoporosis at the baseline DEXA scan or who experience cancer therapy–induced bone loss during ADT should be treated with oral bisphosphonate therapy according to the National Osteoporosis Foundation (2003).

Another significant morbidity that patients with HRPC can develop is bone metastases. Zoledronic acid has demonstrated significant reduction in skeletal morbidity compared with placebo (Saad et al., 2004). Although the main action of zoledronic acid is inhibition of osteoclastic bone resorption, Brubaker, Brown, Vessella, and Corey (2006) reported evidence suggesting direct antitumor effects of zoledronic acid as well as a possible synergism with taxanes.

Adverse Effects of Bisphosphonate Therapy

Long-term use of zoledronic acid has been associated with renal insufficiency and development of osteonecrosis of the jaw (ONJ) (Novartis Pharmaceuticals Corp., 2005). Monitoring for renal insufficiency during zoledronic acid therapy requires assessment of serum creatinine at baseline and before each dose. Dose adjustments are advised for patients whose baseline creatinine clearance is 60 ml/min or less (Novartis Pharmaceuticals Corp.).

ONJ results from temporary or permanent loss of blood supply to the mandible or maxilla. Trauma or damage to the blood vessels that supply blood to the bones, hypercoagulable states, or vasculitis can cause the condition. The loss of blood supply causes minute bone fractures, with ultimate bone collapse

Table 5-7. Pharmacologic Treatments for Erectile Dysfunction

Generic Name	Side Effects	Strengths Available/ Dosing Information	Comments
Sildenafil	Headache Flushing Dyspepsia Nasal congestion Temporary loss of blue-green color discrimination Blue tint to vision Priapism	25 mg, 50 mg, 100 mg Recommended dose is 50 mg, taken as needed, 30–60 minutes before sexual activity. Maximum dosing is once per day. Should be taken on empty stomach	Risk for nonarteritic anterior ischemic optic neuropathy; can cause vision loss 24–36 hours after drug ingestion (Pomeranz & Bhavsar, 2005)
Tadalafil	Headache Flushing Dyspepsia Nasal congestion Back pain, myalgia Priapism	5 mg, 10 mg, 20 mg Recommended starting dose is 10 mg, taken 30–60 minutes before sexual activity Maximum dosing is once per day. Can be taken with or without food	Longer half-life than sildenafil Effective from 30 minutes to 36 hours after ingestion
Vardenafil	Headache Flushing Dyspepsia Myalgia/arthralgia Nasal congestion Temporary loss of blue-green color discrimination Blue tint to vision Priapism	2.5 mg, 5 mg, 10 mg, 20 mg Recommended starting dose is 10 mg, taken 15–30 minutes before sexual activity. Maximum dosing is once per day. Can be taken with or without food	Rapid onset of action (approximately 16 minutes)

Note. Based on information from Bayer Pharmaceuticals Corp., 2003; Eli Lilly & Co., 2008; Pfizer Inc., 2006b; Pomeranz & Bhavsar, 2005; Raina et al., 2004.

Table 5-8. Mechanical Treatments for Erectile Dysfunction

Treatment	Procedure/Guidelines	Side Effects	Comments
Vacuum constriction device (penile pump)	Does not require a prescription. Fit cylinder over lubricated penis. Use hand pump to create vacuum. Pump gently to avoid tissue damage. After erection is achieved, slide constriction band over base of penis and remove pump. Constriction band can remain in place up to 30 minutes. Remove constriction band after sexual intercourse.	Penile petechiae Sensations of numbness (male) or coldness of the penis (partner) Pain or bruising of the penis A sense of trapped semen during ejaculation or delayed ejaculation	The addition of sildenafil may increase rigidity and duration of erection (Raina et al., 2005).
Urethral suppository, synthetic prostaglandin (PGE₁) Alprostadil	Urethral insertion of a pellet containing alprostadil Dose is 125–1,000 mcg, 5–10 minutes before sexual activity. No more than two pellets should be used within a 24-hour period. Patients should urinate before insertion of the pellet, as the drug is designed to dissolve in the residual urine in the urethra. **Contraindications:** Hypersensitivity to alprostadil; abnormal penile anatomy such as urethral stricture; sickle-cell anemia or sickle-cell trait; thrombocytopenia; polycythemia; or multiple myeloma; history of deep vein thrombosis; hyperviscosity syndrome	Syncope Urethral burning sensation Urethral bleeding Urethral pain Hypotension in 3% of patients on first dose	Impairs spontaneity because of the short onset of action If partner is pregnant, a latex condom must be used to prevent fetal exposure to drug

(Continued on next page)

Treatment	Procedure/Guidelines	Side Effects	Comments
Intracavernosal injection of synthetic prostaglandin (PGE₁) Alprostadil	Dose ranges from 2.5–60 mcg, 5–10 minutes before sexual activity. Dose should be slowly titrated to effect. No more than one dose in 24 hours, and no more than 3 doses per week. Drug is effective for up to one hour. Once drug has been injected, manual pressure should be applied to the site for about five minutes to reduce the risk of hematoma formation.	Penile pain Injection site hematoma Dizziness Hypotension Prolonged erections and priapism Development of fibrotic plaques known as corporal fibrosis	
Constriction loop ACTIS® (Vivus, Inc.)	Improves erections by increasing the fullness and firmness of the penis. Tension should be maintained for no more than 30 minutes. Use the least constrictive tension that will maintain an erection. Frequent use or excessive tension of the device may result in bruising of the skin of the penis. Allow 60 minutes between uses. Do not use while under the influence of alcohol or sedatives. Do not fall asleep with device in place. **Contraindications:** Latex allergy Sickle-cell disease Conditions that result in easy bruising or bleeding	Hypersensitivity reaction (latex) Bruising of penis Penile pain	It was designed for the treatment of erectile dysfunction caused by veno-occlusive dysfunction (venous leak).
Penile implant (surgical)	Noninflatable prosthesis, or semirigid rod prosthesis, that involves two bendable rods that are inserted into the corpora cavernosa, allowing the patient to bend the penis into position prior to intercourse. Inflatable penile prosthesis or implant allows for more natural flaccidity and erection, consists of two inflatable rods placed into the corpora cavernosa that are connected to a pump-reservoir. When activated, the device pumps saline from the reservoir into the inflatable rods, resulting in an erection.	Device has the appearance of a permanent erection. Surgical risks of infection, bleeding, pain	Expensive procedures May cause irreversible damage to the penis

Table 5-8. Mechanical Treatments for Erectile Dysfunction *(Continued)*

Note. Based on information from Brown, 2006; Katz, 2005; Mayo Clinic, 2007; Pharmacia and Upjohn Co., 2003; Vivus, Inc., 2001, 2003; Weeks & Ficorelli, 2006b.

(Cope, 2005). The exact incidence of ONJ in patients with cancer is unknown (Novartis Pharmaceuticals Corp., 2005). Risk factors for ONJ among patients with cancer include trauma; advanced age; combination cancer treatment with chemotherapy, RT, or steroid therapy; metastatic disease; blood dyscrasia, anemia, or, coagulopathy; surgical dental procedures; alcohol or tobacco use; and previous bone infection. Studies suggest that approximately 80% of patients with ONJ had undergone dental extraction prior to development of ONJ (Marx, 2003). Patients who have been receiving bisphosphonates for more than six months are at the highest risk for ONJ. In addition, ONJ occurs predominantly in patients receiving the more potent nitrogen-containing IV bisphosphonates rather than the less potent oral bisphosphonate, alendronate (Ruggiero, Mehrotra, Rosenberg, & Engroff, 2004). Postmarketing reports of these

serious bisphosphonate side effects have prompted researchers to study the efficacy of decreased frequency of bisphosphonate administration. Michaelson et al. (2007) demonstrated that a single annual 4 mg dose of zoledronic acid in osteoporotic men on ADT with nonmetastatic disease increased BMD after one year by 4% versus a 3.1% loss in the placebo arm. Current clinical practice guidelines endorse the use of zoledronic acid every three to four weeks in men with bone metastases from prostate cancer (NCCN, 2008); whether a reduced frequency can be appropriate in the metastatic setting will need to be proved in randomized clinical trials.

Assessment

Because of the risk of ONJ, baseline assessment for patients beginning bisphosphonate therapy should include obtaining a history of prior dental procedures and use of dentures, along with an examination of the patient's oral cavity, noting any signs of inflammation or exposed bone (Reilly, 2007). For patients on bisphosphonate therapy who are at risk for ONJ, education concerning dental hygiene and prompt evaluation of any dental or oral lesions are vitally important. Patients beginning bisphosphonate therapy should be reminded that a complete oral and dental examination and all invasive procedures must be completed before beginning bisphosphonate therapy. Nurses can facilitate referral to a dental oncologist or an oral maxillofacial surgeon if a patient reports symptoms of ONJ (Reilly).

IV bisphosphonates have been associated with a decline in renal function; therefore, baseline serum creatinine and creatinine clearance must be evaluated prior to initiation of bisphosphonate therapy. Zoledronic acid should be administered over no less than 15 minutes and no less frequently than every three or four weeks. Serum creatinine must be monitored throughout zoledronic therapy. For patients with creatinine clearance greater than 60 ml/min, the recommended dose remains 4 mg IV over 15 minutes. For patients with reduced creatinine clearance, dosing is calculated to achieve the same area under the curve as in patients with creatinine clearance of 75 ml/min; a dose modification table is available in the drug package insert. Dose interruption is recommended when renal deterioration is noted, which is defined as follows.

- Normal baseline creatinine (< 1.4 mg/ml), increase ≥ 0.5 mg/dl
- Abnormal baseline creatinine (> 1.4 mg/ml), increase ≥ 1 mg/dl

Reinitiate treatment at the same dose received prior to treatment interruption when serum creatinine returns to within 10% of baseline (Novartis Pharmaceuticals Corp., 2005).

Side Effect Management

Common minor side effects of bisphosphonate therapy include transient arthralgia and low-grade fever. Arthralgia is most likely to occur with the first infusion, although some patients may experience persistent arthralgia for the duration of therapy. Some will experience flu-like symptoms, including arthralgia, myalgia, and low-grade fever. A variety of medications can be used to decrease symptoms. Acetaminophen can be given as a premedication to patients with a significant amount of bone metastases, and the patient can be instructed to continue acetaminophen for the next 24 hours. NSAIDs or intermittent steroids also can be used to control discomfort. Additionally, NSAIDs provide analgesic benefit (Martin, 2004). Nonpharmacologic interventions for arthralgia include mild exercise, hydrotherapy, relaxation therapy, application of heat, and massage.

Conclusion

Oncology nurses play a key role in caring for men with prostate cancer and in educating patients and partners, families, and other caregivers in the disease process, treatment options, and associated side effects. Management of treatment-related side effects is an integral part of oncology nursing throughout the continuum of care and will ensure optimal outcomes and QOL. Northouse et al. (2007) assessed 263 patient/spouse dyads with respect to QOL, appraisal of illness, resources, symptoms, and risk for distress across three phases of prostate cancer: newly diagnosed, biochemical recurrence, and advanced. The researchers found that patterns of distress shifted depending on the phase of prostate cancer, and they recommended that phase-specific programs of care are needed to assist both men with prostate cancer and their spouses in managing the effects of illness. Oncology APNs who are charged with development of patient education programs for staff and clinic nurses would be well advised to design disease phase–based teaching tools. Prostate cancer has a varied and often lengthy course, facilitating long-term patient and family relationships that embody trust, mutual respect, and comfort. Living with prostate cancer means living with uncertainty and the effects of treatment: incontinence, ED, hot flashes, and chemotherapy side effects. Only the patient can state whether he is "living well" with prostate cancer.

References

Ahmed, S., & Davies, J. (2005). Managing the complications of prostate cryosurgery. *BJU International, 95*(4), 480–481.

Ahmed, S., Lindsey, B., & Davies, J. (2005). Salvage cryosurgery for locally recurrent prostate cancer following radiotherapy. *Prostate Cancer and Prostatic Disease, 8*(1), 31–35.

Alibhai, S.M.H., Leach, M., Tomlinson, G., Krahn, M.D., Fleshner, N., Holowaty, E., et al. (2005). 30-day mortality and major complications after radical prostatectomy: Influence of age and comorbidity. *Journal of the National Cancer Institute, 97*(20), 1525–1532.

American Society of Anesthesiologists Task Force on Acute Pain Management. (2004). Practice guidelines for acute pain management in the perioperative setting: An updated report. *Anesthesiology, 100*(6), 1573–1581.

Amersham Healthcare. (1998). Metastron [Package insert]. Retrieved August 1, 2007, from http://patient.cancerconsultants.com/druginserts/Strontium_89.pdf

Annon, J.S. (1976). The PLISSIT model: A proposed conceptual scheme for the behavioral treatment of sexual problems. *Journal of Sex Education and Therapy, 2*(2), 1–15.

Balducci, L., & Ershler, W.B. (2005). Cancer and ageing: A nexus at several levels. *Nature Reviews: Cancer, 5*(8), 655–662.

Barnett, J.S. (2005). An emerging role for nurse practitioners— preoperative assessment. *AORN Journal, 82*(5), 825–834.

Barry, M.J., Fowler, F.J., O'Leary, M.P., Bruskewitz, R.C., Holtgrewe, H.L., Mebust, W.K., et al. (1992). The American Urological Association symptom index for benign prostatic hyperplasia: The measurement committee of the American Urological Association. *Journal of Urology, 148*(5), 1549–1557.

Bayer Pharmaceuticals Corp. (2003). Levitra [Package insert]. Retrieved September 1, 2007, from http://www.fda.gov/CDER/foi/label/2003/021400lbl.pdf

Behrend, S.W. (2005). Radiation treatment planning. In C.H. Yarbro, M.H. Frogge, & M. Goodman (Eds.), *Cancer nursing: Principles and practice* (6th ed., pp. 250–282). Sudbury, MA: Jones and Bartlett.

Berry, D. (2007). *Personal patient profile—prostate (P4): A randomized, multi-site trial.* Retrieved August 18, 2007, from http://www.medical.washington.edu/studies/study_details.asp?study=6270

Berthold, D.R., Sternberg, C.N., & Tannock, I.F. (2005). Management of advanced prostate cancer after first-line chemotherapy. *Journal of Clinical Oncology, 23*(32), 8247–8252.

Boccardo, F., Rubagotti, A., Battaglia, M., Di Tonno, P., Selvaggi, F.P., & Conti, G. (2005). Evaluation of tamoxifen and anastrozole in the prevention of gynecomastia and breast pain induced by bicalutamide monotherapy of prostate cancer. *Journal of Clinical Oncology, 23*(4), 808–815.

Boehmer, D., Maingon, P., Poortmans, P., Baron, M.H., Miralbell, R., Remouchamps, V., et al. (2006). Guidelines for primary radiotherapy of patients with prostate cancer. *Radiotherapy and Oncology, 79*(3), 259–269.

Bokhour, B.G., Clark, J.A., Inui, T.S., Silliman, R.A., & Talcott, J.A. (2001). Sexuality after treatment for early prostate cancer: Exploring the meanings of "erectile dysfunction." *Journal of General Internal Medicine, 16*(10), 649–655.

Brown, D.A. (2006). The management of erectile dysfunction and identification of barriers to treatment. *U.S. Pharmacist, 31*(8), 53–64. Retrieved September 4, 2007, from http://www.uspharmacist.com/index.asp?show=article&page=8_1818.htm

Brubaker, K.D., Brown, L.G., Vessella, R.L., & Corey, E. (2006). Administration of zoledronic acid enhances the effects of docetaxel on growth of prostate cancer in the bone environment. *BMC Cancer, 6,* 15.

Bruchovsky, N., Klotz, L., Crook, J., & Goldenberg, S.L. (2007). Locally advanced prostate cancer: Biochemical results from a prospective phase II study of intermittent androgen suppression for men with evidence of prostate-specific antigen recurrence after radiotherapy. *Cancer, 109*(5), 858–867.

Burt, J., Caelli, K., Moore, K., & Anderson, M. (2005). Radical prostatectomy: Men's experiences and postoperative needs. *Journal of Clinical Nursing, 14*(7), 883–890.

Campbell, K.B., & Braithwaite, S.S. (2004). Hospital management of hyperglycemia. *Clinical Diabetes, 22*(2), 81–88.

Camp-Sorrell, D. (2005). Chemotherapy toxicities and management. In C.H. Yarbro, M.H. Frogge, & M. Goodman (Eds.), *Cancer nursing: Principles and practice* (6th ed., pp. 412–457). Sudbury, MA: Jones and Bartlett.

Castle, E.P., Andrews, P.E., Itano, N., Novicki, D.E., Swanson, S.K., & Ferrigni, R.G. (2005). The male sling for post-prostatectomy incontinence: Mean follow-up of 18 months *Journal of Urology, 173*(5), 1657–1660.

Cattani, F., Vavassori, A., Polo, A., Rondi, E., Cambria, R., Orecchia, R., et al. (2006). Radiation exposure after permanent prostate brachytherapy. *Radiotherapy and Oncology, 79*(1), 65–69.

Cope, D. (2005). Clinical update: A nonhealing fractured mandible. *Clinical Journal of Oncology Nursing, 9*(6), 685–687.

Copeland, G.P., Jones, D., & Walters, M. (1991). POSSUM: A scoring system for surgical audit. *British Journal of Surgery, 78*(3), 355–360.

Cytogen Corp. (2003, September). Quadramet [Package insert]. Retrieved July 31, 2007, from http://www.cytogen.com/professional/quadramet/pi.php

Dahn, J.R., Penedo, E.J., Gonzalez, J.S., Esquiabro, M., Antoni, M.H., Roos, B.A., et al. (2004). Sexual functioning and quality of life after prostate cancer treatment: Considering sexual desire. *Urology, 63*(2), 273–277.

D'Amico, A.V., Denham, J.W., Crook, J., Chen, M.-H., Goldhaber, S.Z., Lamb, D.S., et al. (2007). Influence of androgen suppression therapy for prostate cancer on the frequency and timing of fatal myocardial infarctions. *Journal of Clinical Oncology, 25*(17), 2420–2425.

Davison, B.J., Gleave, M.E., Goldenberg, S.L., Degner, L.F., Hoffart, D., & Berkowitz, J. (2002). Assessing information and decision preferences of men with prostate cancer and their partners. *Cancer Nursing, 25*(1), 42–49.

Dawson, N.A. (2007). Epothilones in prostate cancer: Review of clinical experience. *Annals of Oncology, 18*(Suppl. 5), v22–v27.

de Souza Fede, A.B, Bensi, C.G., Trufelli, D.C., de Oliveira Campos, M.P., Pecoroni, P.G., Ranzatti, R.P., et al. (2007). Multivitamins do not improve radiation therapy-related fatigue: Results of a double-blind randomized crossover trial. *American Journal of Clinical Oncology, 30*(4), 432–436.

Diaz, M., & Patterson, S.G. (2004). Management of androgen-independent prostate cancer. *Cancer Control, 11*(6), 364–373.

Dipaola, R.S., Manola, J., Li, S., Vaughn, D., Roth, B., & Wilding, G. (2004). A randomized phase II trial of mitoxantrone, estramustine and vinorelbine or 13-cis retinoic acid, interferon and paclitaxel in patients with metastatic hormone refractory prostate cancer: Results of ECOG 3899. *Journal of Clinical Oncology, 22*(Suppl. 14), Abstract No. 4594. Retrieved July 12, 2008, from http://meeting.ascopubs.org/cgi/content/abstract/22/14_suppl/4594

Dobs, A., & Darkes, M.J. (2005). Incidence and management of gynecomastia in men treated for prostate cancer. *Journal of Urology, 174*(5), 1737–1742.

Docherty, A., Brothwell, P.D., & Symons, M. (2007). The impact of inadequate knowledge on patient and spouse experience of prostate cancer. *Cancer Nursing, 30*(1), 58–63.

Eli Lilly & Co. (2008). Cialis [Package insert]. Retrieved July 15, 2008, from http://pi.lilly.com/us/cialis-pi.pdf

Esmaeli, B., & Hortobagyi, G.N. (2001). Canalicular stenosis as the underlying mechanism for epiphora in patients receiving weekly docetaxel. *Oncologist, 6*(6), 551–552.

Esmaeli, B., Valero, V., Ahmadi, A., & Booser, D. (2001). Canalicular stenosis secondary to docetaxel (Taxotere): A newly recognized side effect. *Ophthalmology, 108*(5), 994–995.

Eymard, J.C., Priou, F., Zannetti, A., Ravaud, A., Lepille, D., Kerbrat, P., et al. (2007). Randomized phase II study of docetaxel plus estramustine and single-agent docetaxel in patients with metastatic hormone-refractory prostate cancer. *Annals of Oncology, 18*(6), 1064–1070.

Ficorelli, C.T., & Weeks, B. (2006). Facing up to prostate cancer. *Nursing, 36*(5), 66–68.

Gallagher, E., & Gapstur, R. (2006). Hormone-refractory prostate cancer: A shifting paradigm in treatment. *Clinical Journal of Oncology Nursing, 10*(2), 233–240.

Giarelli, E., McCorkle, R., & Monturo, C. (2003). Caring for a spouse after prostate surgery: The preparedness needs of wives. *Journal of Family Nursing, 9*(4), 453–485.

Goodin, S., Medina, P., Capanna, T., Shih, W.J., Abraham, S., Winnie, J., et al. (2005). Effect of docetaxel in patients with hormone-dependent prostate-specific antigen progression after local therapy for prostate cancer. *Journal of Clinical Oncology, 23*(15), 3352–3357.

Gosney, M. (2005). Clinical assessment of elderly people with cancer. *Lancet Oncology, 6*(10), 790–797.

Griffin, A.D., & O'Rourke, M.E. (2001). Expectant management of prostate cancer. *Seminars in Oncology Nursing, 17*(2), 101–107.

Guise, T.A. (2006). Bone loss and fracture risk associated with cancer therapy. *Oncologist, 11*(10), 1121–1131.

Han, K.R., & Belldegrun, A.S. (2004). Third-generation cryosurgery for primary and recurrent prostate cancer. *BJU International, 93*(1), 14–18.

Held-Warmkessel, J. (2005). Prostate cancer. In C.H. Yarbro, M.H. Frogge, & M. Goodman (Eds.), *Cancer nursing: Principles and practice* (6th ed., pp. 1552–1580). Sudbury, MA: Jones and Bartlett.

Hollenbeck, B.K., Dunn, R.L., Wei, J.T., Montie, J.E., & Sanda, M.G. (2003). Determinants of long-term sexual health outcome after radical prostatectomy measured by a validated instrument. *Journal of Urology, 169*(4), 1453–1457.

Hunter, K.F., Moore, K.N., & Glazener, C.M. (2007). Conservative management for postprostatectomy urinary incontinence. *Cochrane Database of Systematic Reviews* 2007, Issue 1. Art. No.: CD001843. DOI: 10.1002/14651858.CD001843.pub3.

Hussain, M., Faulkner, J., Vaishampayan, U., Lara, P., Petrylak, D., Colevas, D., et al. (2004). Epothilone B (Epo-B) analogue BMS-247550 (NSC #710428) administered every 21 days in patients (pts) with hormone refractory prostate cancer (HRPC). A Southwest Oncology Group Study (S0111). *Journal of Clinical Oncology, 22*(Suppl. 14), Abstract No. 4510. Retrieved July 11, 2008, from http://meeting.ascopubs.org/cgi/content/abstract/22/14_suppl/4510

Immunex Corp. (2002). Novantrone [Package insert]. Retrieved August 30, 2007, from http://www.fda.gov/MEDWATCH/SAFETY/2003/03Jan_labels/novantrone.pdf

Incrocci, L. (2006). Sexual function after external-beam radiotherapy for prostate cancer: What do we know? *Critical Reviews in Oncology Hematology, 57*(2), 165–173.

Ingram, S.S., Sea, P.H., Martell, R.E., Clipp, E.C., Doyle, M.E., Montana, G.S., et al. (2002). Comprehensive assessment of the elderly cancer patient: The feasibility of self-report methodology. *Journal of Clinical Oncology, 20*(3), 770–775.

Iwamoto, R.R., & Maher, K.E. (2001). Radiation therapy for prostate cancer. *Seminars in Oncology Nursing, 17*(2), 90–100.

Johnson, B.K. (2004). Prostate cancer and sexuality: Implications for nursing. *Geriatric Nursing, 25*(6), 341–347.

Kagee, A., Kruus, L.K., Malkowicz, S., Vaughn, D.J., & Coyne, J.C. (2001). The experience of hot flashes among prostate cancer patients receiving hormone therapy. *Proceedings of the American Society of Clinical Oncology, 20,* Abstract No. 2999. Retrieved July 14, 2008, from http://www.asco.org/ASCO/Abstracts+%26+Virtual+Meeting/Abstracts?&vmview=abst_detail_view&confID=10&abstractID=2999

Katz, A. (2005). What happened? Sexual consequences of prostate cancer and its treatment. *Canadian Family Physician, 51,* 977–982.

Katz, A. (2007a). *Breaking the silence on cancer and sexuality: A handbook for healthcare providers.* Pittsburgh, PA: Oncology Nursing Society.

Katz, A. (2007b). Quality of life for men with prostate cancer. *Cancer Nursing, 30*(4), 302–308.

Keating, N.L., O'Malley, A.J., & Smith, M.R. (2006). Diabetes and cardiovascular disease during androgen deprivation therapy for prostate cancer. *Journal of Clinical Oncology, 24*(27), 4448–4456.

Kuck, A.W. (2006, November). Caring for diabetic patients with cancer receiving steroids. *Oncology Nursing Society Nurse Practitioner Special Interest Group Newsletter, 17*(3). Retrieved January 14, 2008, from http://onsopcontent.ons.org/Publications/SIGNewsletters/np/np17.3.html#story6

Lee, A.K., & Frank, S.J. (2006). Update on radiation therapy in prostate cancer. *Hematology/Oncology Clinics of North America, 20*(4), 857–878.

Liepe, K., Runge, R., & Kotzerke, J. (2005). Systemic radionuclide therapy in pain palliation. *American Journal of Hospice and Palliative Care, 22*(6), 457–464.

Litwin, M.S. (2002). *RAND 12-item health survey v2 (SF-12 v2) and UCLA prostate cancer index short form.* Retrieved August 15, 2007, from http://www.uclaurology.com/site_uo/pdf/PCI_short_scoring.pdf

Loeb, S., & Nadler, R.B. (2006). Management of the complications of external beam radiotherapy and brachytherapy. *Current Urology Reports, 7*(3), 200–208.

Loprinzi, C.L., Khoyratty, B.S., Dueck, A., Barton, D.L., Jafar, S., Rowland, K.M., Jr., et al. (2007). Gabapentin for hot flashes in men: NCCTG trial N00CB. *Journal of Clinical Oncology, 25*(Suppl. 18), Abstract No. 9005. Retrieved July 11, 2008, from http://meeting.ascopubs.org/cgi/content/abstract/25/18_suppl/9005

Maas, H.A., Janssen-Heijnen, M.L., Olde Rikkert, M.G., & Machteld, W. (2007). Comprehensive geriatric assessment and its clinical impact in oncology. *European Journal of Cancer, 43*(15), 2161–2169.

Madsen, L.T., & Ganey-Code, E. (2006). Assessing and addressing erectile function concerns in patients postprostatectomy. *Oncology Nursing Forum, 33*(2), 209–211.

Maliski, S.L., Heilemann, M.V., & McCorkle, R. (2002). From "death sentence" to "good cancer": Couples' transformation of a prostate cancer diagnosis. *Nursing Research, 51*(6), 391–397.

Mariani, G., Boni, G., Genovesi, D., Pastina, I., Chioni, A., Pesella, F., Cianci, C., et al. (2006). Early response and toxicity of ^{153}Sm-EDTMP combined with docetaxel in patients with hormone-refractory metastatic prostate cancer. *Journal of Nuclear Medicine, 47*(Suppl. 1), 104P.

Martin, V.R. (2004). Arthralgias and myalgias. In C.H. Yarbro, M.H. Frogge, & M. Goodman (Eds.), *Cancer symptom management* (3rd ed., pp. 17–28). Sudbury, MA: Jones and Bartlett.

Marx, R.E. (2003). Pamidronate (Aredia) and zoledronate (Zometa) induced avascular necrosis of the jaws: A growing epidemic. *Journal of Oral and Maxillofacial Surgery, 61*(9), 1115–1117.

Mathis, A.S., & Liu, M.T. (2005). Corticosteroids: An important cause of hyperglycemia. *American Journal of Health-System Pharmacy, 62*(19), 1976–1979.

Mayo Clinic. (2007, August). *Penis pumps for erectile dysfunction: Improve your sexual function.* Retrieved July 15, 2008, from http://www.mayoclinic.com/health/penispump/MC00059

McGuire, D.B. (2004). Occurrence of cancer pain. *Journal of the National Cancer Institute Monographs, 2004*(32), 52–56.

McGuire, E.J. (2005). Urinary incontinence: A diverse condition. *Journal of Urology, 173*(5), 1453–1454.

McLeod, D.G., Iversen, P., See, W.A., Morris, T., Armstrong, J., & Wirth, M.P. (2006). Bicalutamide 150 mg plus standard care vs standard care alone for early prostate cancer. *BJU International, 97*(2), 247-254.

Merrick, G.S., Butler, W.M., & Wallner, K.E. (2005). Brachytherapy-associated erectile dysfunction. *Current Sexual Health Reports, 2*(1/2), 21–26.

Michaelson, M.D., Kaufman, D.S., Lee, H., McGovern, F.J., Kantoff, P.W., Fallon, M.A., et al. (2007). Randomized controlled trial of annual zoledronic acid to prevent gonadotropin-releasing hormone agonist-induced bone loss in men with prostate cancer. *Journal of Clinical Oncology, 25*(9), 1038–1042.

Michalski, J., Mutic, S., Eichling, J., & Ahmed, S.N. (2003). Radiation exposure to family and household members after prostate brachytherapy. *International Journal of Radiation Oncology, Biology, Physics, 56*(3), 764–768.

Montorsi, F., Maga, T., Strambi, L.F., Salonia, A., Barbieri, L., Scattoni, V., et al. (2000). Sildenafil taken at bedtime significantly increases nocturnal erections: Results of a placebo-controlled study. *Urology, 56*(6), 906–911.

Moore, K.N., Truong, V., Estey, E., & Voaklander, D.C. (2007). Urinary incontinence after radical prostatectomy: Can men at risk be identified preoperatively? *Journal of Wound, Ostomy and Continence Nursing, 34*(3), 270–279.

Moore, S. (2004). Menopausal symptoms. In C.H. Yarbro, M.H. Frogge, & M. Goodman (Eds.), *Cancer symptom management* (3rd ed., pp. 571–590). Sudbury, MA: Jones and Bartlett.

Nakabayashi, M., Bartlett, R.A., & Oh, W.K. (2006). Treatment of bicalutamide-induced gynecomastia with breast-reduction surgery in prostate cancer. *Journal of Clinical Oncology, 24*(18), 2958–2959.

National Cancer Institute. (2007a). *Clinical trials: Prostate cancer.* Retrieved August 20, 2007, from http://www.cancer.gov/search/ResultsClinicalTrialsAdvanced.aspx?protocolsearchid=4372165

National Cancer Institute. (2007b). *PCOS data collection.* Retrieved August 15, 2007, from http://healthservices.cancer.gov/pcos/data.html

National Cancer Institute. (2007c). *Prostate cancer (PDQ®): Health professional version.* Retrieved July 20, 2007, from http://www.cancer.gov/cancertopics/pdq/treatment/prostate/healthprofessional/allpages

National Cancer Institute Cancer Therapy Evaluation Program. (2006). *Common terminology criteria for adverse events* (Version 3.0). Retrieved August 11, 2007, from http://ctep.cancer.gov/forms/CTCAEv3.pdf

National Comprehensive Cancer Network. (2008). *NCCN Clinical Practice Guidelines in Oncology™. Prostate cancer* [v.1.2008]. Retrieved July 11, 2008, from http://www.nccn.org/professionals/physician_gls/PDF/prostate.pdf

National Osteoporosis Foundation. (2003). *Physician's guide to prevention and treatment of osteoporosis.* Retrieved July 14, 2008, from http://www.guideline.gov/summary/summary.aspx?doc_id=3862

Navon, L., & Morag, A. (2003). Advanced prostate cancer patients' relationships with their spouses following hormonal therapy. *European Journal of Oncology Nursing, 7*(2), 73–80.

Nilsson, S., Franzen, L., Parker, C., Tyrrell, C., Blom, R., Tennvall, J., et al. (2007). Bone-targeted radium-223 in symptomatic, hormone-refractory prostate cancer: A randomised, multicentre, placebo-controlled phase II study. *Lancet Oncology, 8*(7), 587–594.

Nitti, V., Kim, Y., & Combs, A.J. (1994). Correlation of the AUA symptom index with urodynamics in patients with suspected benign prostatic hyperplasia. *Neurourology and Urodynamics, 13*(5), 521–529.

Northouse, L.L., Mood, D.W., Montie, J.E., Sandler, H.M., Forman, J.D., Hussain, M., et al. (2007). Living with prostate cancer: Patients' and spouses' psychosocial status and quality of life. *Journal of Clinical Oncology, 25*(27), 4171–4177.

Novartis Pharmaceuticals Corp. (2005). Zometa [Package insert]. Retrieved August 2, 2007, from http://www.pharma.us.novartis.com/product/pi/pdf/Zometa.pdf

Ohebshalom, M., Parker, M., Guhring, P., & Mulhall, J.P. (2005). The efficacy of sildenafil citrate following radiation therapy for prostate cancer: Temporal considerations. *Journal of Urology, 174*(1), 258–262.

Ornish, D., Weidner, G., Fair, W.R., Marlin, R., Pettengill, E.B., Raisin, C.J., et al. (2005). Intensive lifestyle changes may affect the progression of prostate cancer. *Journal of Urology, 174*(3), 1065–1070.

Paice, J.A. (2004). Pain. In C.H. Yarbro, M.H. Frogge, & M. Goodman (Eds.), *Cancer symptom management* (3rd ed., pp. 77–93). Sudbury, MA: Jones and Bartlett.

Palmer, M.H., Fogarty, L.A., Somerfield, M.R., & Powel, L.L. (2003). Incontinence after prostatectomy: Coping with incontinence after prostate cancer surgery. *Oncology Nursing Forum, 30*(2), 229–238.

Pandit, M.K., Burke, J., Gustafson, A.B., Minocha, A., & Peiris, A.N. (1993). Drug-induced disorders of glucose tolerance. *Annals of Internal Medicine, 118*(7), 529–539.

Paterson, J. (2000). Stigma associated with postprostatectomy urinary incontinence. *Journal of Wound, Ostomy, and Continence Nursing, 27*(3), 168–173.

Penson, D.F., Chan, J.M., & Urologic Diseases in America Project. (2007). Prostate cancer. *Journal of Urology, 177*(6), 2020–2029.

Penson, D.F., McLerran, D., Feng, Z., Li, L., Albertsen, P.C., Gilliland, F.D., et al. (2005). 5-year urinary and sexual outcomes after radical prostatectomy: Results from the prostate cancer outcomes study. *Journal of Urology, 173*(5), 1701–1705.

Perdona, S., Autorino, R., De Placido, S., D'Armiento, M., Gallo, A., Damiano, R., et al. (2005). Efficacy of tamoxifen and radiotherapy for prevention and treatment of gynaecomastia and breast pain caused by bicalutamide in prostate cancer: A randomized controlled trial. *Lancet Oncology, 6*(5), 295–300.

PerkinElmer, Inc. (2007). *Phosphorus-32 handling precautions.* Retrieved July 15, 2008, from http://las.perkinelmer.com/content/TechnicalInfo/TCH_Phosphorus32.pdf

Petrylak, D.P., Tangen, C.M., Hussain, M.H.A., Lara, P.N., Jr., Jones, J.A., Taplin, M.E., et al. (2004). Docetaxel and estramustine compared with mitoxantrone and prednisone for advanced refractory prostate cancer. *New England Journal of Medicine, 351*(15), 1513–1520.

Pfizer Inc. (2006a). Estramustine [Package insert]. Retrieved July 31, 2007, from http://www.pfizer.com/pfizer/download/uspi_emcyt.pdf

Pfizer Inc. (2006b). Viagra [Package insert]. Retrieved September 1, 2007, from http://www.pfizer.com/pfizer/download/uspi_viagra.pdf

Pharmacia and Upjohn Co. (2003). Caverject impulse [Package insert]. Retrieved September 4, 2007, from http://www.pfizer.com/pfizer/download/uspi_caverject_impulse.pdf

Pietrzak, P., Arya, M., & Patel, H.R. (2006). Anti-emetic therapy: Updating urological cancer-care providers. *BJU International, 97*(4), 673–675.

Polovich, M., White, J.M., & Kelleher, L.O. (Eds.). (2005). *Chemotherapy and biotherapy guidelines and recommendations for practice* (2nd ed., pp. 233–234). Pittsburgh, PA: Oncology Nursing Society.

Pomeranz, H., & Bhavsar, A. (2005). Nonarteritic ischemic optic neuropathy developing soon after use of sildenafil (Viagra): A report of seven new cases. *Journal of Neuro-Ophthalmology, 25*(1), 9–13.

Potosky, A.L., Reeve, B.B., Clegg, L.X., Hoffman, R.M., Stephenson, R.A., Albertsen, P.C., et al. (2002). Quality of life following localized prostate cancer treated initially with androgen deprivation therapy or no therapy. *Journal of the National Cancer Institute, 94*(6), 430–437.

Pound, C.R., Partin, A.W., Eisenberger, M.A., Chan, D.W., Pearson, J.D., & Walsh, P.C. (1999). Natural history of progression after PSA elevation following radical prostatectomy. *JAMA, 281*(17), 1591–1597.

Prayer-Galetti, T., Sacco, E., Pagano, F., Gardiman, M., Cisternino, A., Betto, G., et al. (2007). Long-term follow-up of a neoadjuvant chemohormonal taxane-based phase II trial before radical prostatectomy in patients with non-metastatic high-risk prostate cancer. *BJU International, 100*(2), 274–280.

Prezioso, D., Piccirillo, G., Galasso, R., Altieri, V., Mirone, V., & Lotti, T. (2004). Gynecomastia due to hormone therapy for advanced prostate cancer: A report of ten surgically treated cases and a review of treatment options. *Tumori, 90*(4), 410–415.

Raina, R., Agarwal, A., Allamaneni, S.S., Lakin, M.M., & Zippe, C.D. (2005). Sildenafil citrate and vacuum constriction device combination enhances sexual satisfaction in erectile dysfunction after radical prostatectomy. *Urology, 65*(2), 360–364.

Raina, R., Lakin, M.M., Agarwal, A., Mascha, M., Montague, D.K., Klein, E., et al. (2004). Efficacy and factors associated with successful outcome of sildenafil citrate use for erectile dysfunction after radical prostatectomy. *Urology, 63*(5), 960–966.

Ramanathan, T.S., Moppett, I.K., Wenn, R., & Moran, C.G. (2005). POSSUM scoring for patients with fractured neck of femur. *British Journal of Anaesthesia, 94*(4), 430–433.

Rao, A.V., Seo, P.H., & Cohen, H.J. (2004). Geriatric assessment and comorbidity. *Seminars in Oncology, 31*(2), 149–159.

Reilly, M.M. (2007). Osteonecrosis of the jaw in a patient receiving bisphosphonate therapy. *Oncology Nursing Forum, 34*(2), 301–305.

Rosen, R.C., Althof, S.E., & Giuliano, F. (2006). Research instruments for the diagnosis and treatment of patients with erectile dysfunction. *Urology, 68*(Suppl. 3), 6–16.

Rosen, R.C., Cappelleri, J.C., Smith, M.D., Lipsky, J., & Pena, B.M. (1999). Development and evaluation of an abridged, 5-item version of the International Index of Erectile Function (IIEF-5) as a diagnostic tool for erectile dysfunction. *International Journal of Impotence Research, 11*(6), 319–326.

Ross, R.W., & Small, E.J. (2002). Osteoporosis in men treated with androgen deprivation therapy for prostate cancer. *Journal of Urology, 167*(5), 1952–1956.

Rubenstein, L.Z. (2004). Comprehensive geriatric assessment: From miracle to reality. *Journal of Gerontology, 59A*, 473–477.

Ruggiero, S.L., Mehrotra, B., Rosenberg, T.J., & Engroff, S.L. (2004). Osteonecrosis of the jaws associated with the use of bisphosphonates: A review of 63 cases. *Journal of Oral and Maxillofacial Surgery, 62*(5), 527–534.

Saad, F., Gleason, D.M., Murray, R., Tchekmedyian, S., Venner, P., Lacombe, L., et al. (2004). Long-term efficacy of zoledronic acid for the prevention of skeletal complications in patients with metastatic hormone-refractory prostate cancer. *Journal of the National Cancer Institute, 96*(11), 879–882.

Sanofi-Aventis. (2003). Taxotere [Package insert]. Retrieved August 30, 2007, from http://www.usrf.org/news/19MAY04taxotere/Taxotere%20Pkg%20Insert.pdf

Sartor, A.O., Reid, R., Higano, C., Bushnell, D., & Quick, D. (2005). Repeated dose samarium 153 lexidronam in patients with prostate cancer bone metastases. *Journal of Clinical Oncology, 23*(Suppl. 16), Abstract No. 4635. Retrieved July 12, 2008 from http://meeting.ascopubs.org/cgi/content/abstract/23/16_suppl/4635

Savoie, M., Kim, S.S., & Soloway, M.S. (2003). A prospective study measuring penile length in men treated with radical prostatectomy for prostate cancer. *Journal of Urology, 169*(4), 1462–1464.

Schulmeister, L. (2005). Article on mitoxantrone-induced extravasation raised useful questions [Letter to the editor]. *Oncology Nursing Forum, 32*(4), 719–721.

See, W.A., Wirth, M.P., McLeod, D.G., Iversen, P., Klimberg, I., Gleason, D., et al. (2002). Bicalutamide as immediate therapy either alone or as adjuvant to standard care of patients with localized or locally advanced prostate cancer: First analysis of the early prostate cancer program. *Journal of Urology, 168*(2), 429–435.

Serber, W., Brady, L.W., Zhang, M., & Hoppe, R.T. (2004). Radiation treatment of benign disease. In C.A. Perez, L.W. Brady, E.C. Halperin, & R.K. Schmidt-Ullrich (Eds.), *Principles and practice of radiation oncology* (4th ed., pp. 2332–2351). Philadelphia: Lippincott Williams & Wilkins.

Shabsigh, R. (2004). Therapy for ED: PDE-5 inhibitors. *Endocrine, 23*(2–3), 135–141.

Shahinian, V.B., Kuo, Y.F., Freeman, J.L., & Goodwin, J.S. (2005). Risk of fracture after androgen deprivation for prostate cancer. *New England Journal of Medicine, 352*(2), 154–164.

Sharifi, N., Gulley, J.L., & Dahut, W.L. (2005). Androgen deprivation therapy for prostate cancer. *JAMA, 294*(2), 238–244.

Simon, B.E., Hoffman, S., & Kahn, S. (1973). Classification and surgical correction of gynecomastia. *Plastic and Reconstructive Surgery, 51*(1), 48–52.

Siston, A.K., Knight, S.J., Slimack, N.P., Chmiel, J.S., Nadler, R.B., Lyons, T.M., et al. (2003). Quality of life after a diagnosis of prostate cancer among men of lower socioeconomic status: Results from the Veterans Affairs Cancer of the Prostate Outcomes Study. *Urology, 61*(1), 172–178.

Smathers, S., Wallner, K., Korssjoen, T., Bergsagel, C., Hudson, R.H., Sutlief, S., et al. (1999). Radiation safety parameters following prostate brachytherapy. *International Journal of Radiation Oncology, Biology, Physics, 45*(2), 397–399.

Snow, A.L., & Shuster, J.L., Jr. (2006). Assessment and treatment of persistent pain in persons with cognitive and communicative impairment. *Journal of Clinical Psychology, 62*(11), 1379–1387.

Speight, J.L., & Roach, M., III. (2005). Radiotherapy in the management of clinically localized prostate cancer: Evolving standards, consensus, controversies and new directions. *Journal of Clinical Oncology, 23*(32), 8176–8185.

Stanford, J.L., Feng, Z., Hamilton, A.S., Gilliland, F.D., Stephenson, R.A., Eley, J.W., et al. (2000). Urinary and sexual function after radical prostatectomy for clinically localized prostate cancer: The prostate cancer outcomes study. *JAMA, 283*(3), 354–360.

Sternberg, C.N., Petrylak, D., Witjes, F., Ferrero, J., Eymard, J., Falcon, S., et al. (2007). Satraplatin (S) demonstrates significant clinical benefits for the treatment of patients with HRPC: Results of a randomized phase III trial. *Journal of Clinical Oncology, 25*(Suppl. 18), Abstract No. 5019. Retrieved July 12, 2008, from http://meeting.ascopubs.org/cgi/content/abstract/25/18_suppl/5019

Sternberg, C.N., Whelan, P., Hetherington, J., Paluchowska, B., Slee, P.H., Vekemans, K., et al. (2005). Phase III trial of satraplatin, an oral platinum plus prednisone vs. prednisone alone in patients with hormone-refractory prostate cancer. *Oncology, 68*(1), 2–9.

Stipetich, R.L., Abel, L.J., Anderson, R.L., Butler, W.M., Wallner, K.E., & Merrick, G.S. (2005). Nursing considerations in brachytherapy-related erectile dysfunction. *Urologic Nursing, 25*(4), 249–254.

Stipetich, R.L., Abel, L.J., Blatt, H.J., Galbreath, R.W., Lief, J.H., Butler, W.M., et al. (2002). Nursing assessment of sexual function following permanent prostate brachytherapy for patients with early-stage prostate cancer. *Clinical Journal of Oncology Nursing, 6*(5), 271–274.

Strassels, S.A., McNicol, E., & Suleman, R. (2005). Postoperative pain management: A practical review, part 1. *American Journal of Health-System Pharmacy, 62*(18), 1904–1916.

Su, A.W., & Jani, A.B. (2007). Chronic genitourinary and gastrointestinal toxicity of prostate cancer patients undergoing pelvic radiotherapy with intensity-modulated versus 4-field technique. *American Journal of Clinical Oncology, 30*(3), 215–219.

Tannock, I.F., de Wit, R., Berry, W.R., Horti, J., Pluzanska, A., Chi, K.N., et al. (2004). Docetaxel plus prednisone or mitoxantrone plus prednisone for advanced prostate cancer. *New England Journal of Medicine, 351*(15), 1502–1512.

Tashkandi, M., Al-Qattan, M.M., Hassanain, J.M., Hawary, M.B., & Sultan, M. (2004). The surgical management of high-grade gynecomastia. *Annals of Plastic Surgery, 53*(1), 17–20.

Thompson, C.A., Shanafelt, T.D., & Loprinzi, C.L. (2003). Andropause: Symptom management for prostate cancer patients treated with hormonal ablation. *Oncologist, 8*(5), 474–487.

Tiefer, L., & Schuetz-Mueller, D. (1995). Psychological issues in diagnosis and treatment of erectile disorders. *Urologic Clinics of North America, 22*(4), 767–773.

Tunn, U. (2007). The current status of intermittent androgen deprivation (IAD) therapy for prostate cancer: Putting IAD under the spotlight. *BJU International, 99*(Suppl. 1), 19–22.

Vivus, Inc. (2001). Actis [Package insert]. Retrieved September 1, 2007, from http://www.vivus.com/res/ACTIS_PI_1.3.3.pdf

Vivus, Inc. (2003). Muse [Package insert]. Retrieved September 3, 2007, from http://www.muserx.net/res/pack_inserts_PFI_1.3.pdf

Walton, J., & Sullivan, N. (2004). Men of prayer: Spirituality of men with prostate cancer: A grounded theory study. *Journal of Holistic Nursing, 22*(2), 133–151.

Warlick, C., Trock, B.J., Landis, P., Epstein, J.I., & Carter, H.B. (2006). Delayed versus immediate surgical intervention and prostate cancer outcome. *Journal of the National Cancer Institute, 98*(5), 355–357.

Weeks, B., & Ficorelli, C.T. (2006a). How new drugs help treat erectile dysfunction. *Nursing, 36*(1), 18–19.

Weeks, B., & Ficorelli, C.T. (2006b). Treating erectile dysfunction without first-line drugs. *Nursing, 36*(3), 26–27.

Widmark, A., Fossa, S.D., Lundmo, P., Damber, J.E., Vaage, S., Damber, L., et al. (2003). Does prophylactic breast irradiation prevent antiandrogen-induced gynecomastia? Evaluation of 253 patients in the randomized Scandinavian trial SPCG-7/SFUO-3. *Urology, 61*(1), 145–151.

Wirth, M., See, W.A., II, McLeod, D.G., Iversen, P., Morris, T., & Armstrong, J. (2006). Delaying metastatic disease progression in locally advanced disease: Results from the Early Prostate Cancer Program at a median follow-up of 7.4 years. *Journal of Clinical Oncology, 24*(Suppl. 18), Abstract No. 4629. Retrieved July 10, 2008 from http://meeting.ascopubs.org/cgi/content/abstract/24/18_suppl/4629

Wirth, M., Tyrrell, C., Delaere, K., Sanchez-Chapado, M., Ramon, J., Wallace, D.M., et al. (2005). Bicalutamide ('Casodex') 150 mg in addition to standard care in patients with nonmetastatic prostate cancer: Updated results from a randomized double-blind phase III study (median follow-up 5.1 y) in the early prostate cancer programme. *Prostate Cancer and Prostatic Diseases, 8*(2), 194–200.

World Health Organization. (2007). *WHO's pain ladder.* Retrieved August 17, 2007, from http://www.who.int/cancer/palliative/painladder/en

CHAPTER 6

Survivorship Issues in Prostate Cancer

Cathy Fortenbaugh, RN, MSN, AOCN®

"I gained weight from the hormone treatments and I still have not been able to get it off. The only thing that still really bothers me is the impotence; otherwise, I feel as though I never had cancer."
—Joseph Sickels, a 77-year-old prostate cancer survivor diagnosed in 2002

Introduction

The number of men diagnosed with prostate cancer increased dramatically in the late 1980s and early 1990s. This increase has been attributed to the detection of early-stage disease. During this time, prostate cancer surpassed lung cancer as the number-one noncutaneous cancer diagnosis in men. Improved screening methods, including prostate-specific antigen (PSA) testing, accounts for the largest increase in men being diagnosed with early-stage disease. In turn, this testing has resulted in more men living longer lives with prostate cancer. Researchers expect that 28,660 men will die of prostate cancer in 2008, thus representing a new statistical low. In many instances, prostate cancer can now be considered a chronic disease (American Cancer Society [ACS], 2008; Jemal et al., 2008).

Survivorship is an important part of the cancer continuum that currently is underaddressed. Patients perceive the healthcare team as an important component of their overall support system during the course of treatment. When treatment is complete, patients return to less frequent follow-up care with the oncology team and routine care in the community (Haylock, Mitchell, Cox, Temple, & Curtiss, 2007; Hewitt, Greenfield, & Stovall, 2005). The completion of active treatment is fraught with many emotions and concerns for cancer survivors. The Institute of Medicine (IOM) released a report on cancer survivorship in 2005 titled "From Cancer Patient to Cancer Survivor: Lost in Transition." This report identified the lack of formalized communication between oncology and primary healthcare providers at the conclusion of cancer treatment as a major barrier to the improvement of care of the cancer survivor. The IOM recommended that an individualized post-treatment plan be developed for each patient completing treatment, regardless of the type (Hewitt et al.).

This chapter will focus on survivorship issues related to prostate cancer and the multiple treatment modalities employed to treat the disease. Nursing assessment, interventions, and education for late effects of each modality will be discussed. Late psychosocial effects of treatment and some quality-of-life (QOL) issues are also examined. Finally, palliative care and hospice, in addition to wellness care, for patients with advanced prostate cancer will be explored.

Need for Ongoing Intervention

Assessment

Essential to any post-treatment plan of care is assessment. Patients with cancer tend to neglect or underreport symptoms from treatment unless otherwise prompted to do so (Fortner et al., 2003; Johnson, Moore, & Fortner, 2007; Rutledge & McGuire, 2004; Ward et al., 1993). Routine, systematic assessment allows patients the opportunity to report symptoms upon each office visit, thus enabling oncology practitioners to identify and manage problems appropriately. Ongoing assessment during regularly scheduled intervals is important, as symptoms do not always occur as expected. The use of a standardized grading scale is recommended when assessing treatment-related side effects. Grading scales most frequently cited in the literature include World Health Organization, Radiation Therapy Oncology Group, and the National Cancer Institute (NCI) Common Terminology Criteria for Adverse Events (CTCAE). Consistent use of a standardized assessment tool allows for improved communication among healthcare workers and accurate symptom reporting. In addition, use of a standardized QOL assessment tool may detect functional changes indicative of new or worsening symptomatology or one's decreased ability to cope with changes brought on by a cancer diagnosis or treatment. Practitioners must realize the difference that exists between change in function and the amount of distress the patient is experiencing over such a change (Reeve, Potosky, & Willis, 2006). Ongoing patient assessment includes patient-reported symptoms and severity, functional status, psychosocial status, and evaluation of laboratory values and interpretation of radiologic interventions (Johnson et al.). QOL assessment tools are helpful in gauging a patient's level of distress and are discussed in more detail later in this chapter.

Education

While patient education begins at diagnosis, a key aspect of survivorship is ongoing education, which includes psychological reinforcement and support. Initial treatment decisions have long-term implications. Men with newly diagnosed prostate cancer need to be actively involved in making treatment decisions, most of which have a significant impact on QOL for many years. Patient goals for survivorship should be explored and considered when developing a plan for follow-up care. When treatment is complete, education must include expectations as to what one might experience during the transitional period from treatment completion to follow-up. Issues that should be addressed include

- Late effects—when they might occur, how they should be managed, how long they will last
- Potential psychosocial issues and available support
- Healthy lifestyle changes and ongoing cancer screening.

Survivorship begins upon diagnosis. This concept originated with the founding charter of the National Coalition for Cancer Survivorship (NCCS) in 1986 (Haylock et al., 2007). Unfortunately, some men will be diagnosed with advanced prostate cancer. For these individuals, supportive measures and therapeutic strategies are designed to improve QOL and are a part of survivorship care.

Hormonal Manipulation

Androgen deprivation therapy (ADT) will induce remission in most men (80%–90%) with advanced prostate cancer (Otto, 2004). Remission can last 12–33 months, meaning that some men with advanced disease may be in a state of stable disease for upwards of three years. Many men receive hormonal manipulation for several months or years after attempts at definitive treatment have failed. In addition, hormonal manipulation is used along with external beam radiation therapy (RT), brachytherapy, and radical prostatectomy (Otto). Three major categories of hormonal therapies exist for prostate cancer: luteinizing hormone-releasing hormone agonists, antiandrogens, and nonsteroidal antiandrogens. Long-term

effects depend on the class of medication used. See Table 6-1 for side effect profiles for each class of agent.

In general, long-term side effects most commonly experienced by men undergoing ADT include hot flashes, osteoporosis, erectile dysfunction, fatigue, and weight gain. Unfortunately, no large outcome trials in men on ADT have compared the available therapies for adverse effects. Furthermore, no therapies, as of yet, have been specifically approved for treatment of adverse effects in men on ADT (Guise et al., 2007).

Hot Flashes

The hot flash daily interference scale has been evaluated in breast cancer survivors (Carpenter, 2001) and may be helpful in patients with prostate cancer. When using this tool, the following items are rated on a 0–10 scale: work, social activities, leisure activities, sleep, mood, concentration, relationships with others, sexuality, enjoyment of life, and overall QOL. A score of 0 means no interference, and 10 means the most interference possible (Kattan, 2006). Oncology nurses are likely more familiar with discussing hot flash management with survivors of breast cancer, as a great deal of literature focuses on management of hot flashes in this patient population. However, hot flashes are a common side effect for men undergoing ADT and should be addressed, as they may last for several months. For nonpharmacologic techniques to help men to manage hot flashes, see Figure 6-1.

Pharmacologic interventions that may provide some degree of relief from hot flashes include the use of selective serotonin reuptake inhibitors (SSRIs) including venlafaxine, fluoxetine, and paroxetine (Moore, 2004; Thompson, Shanafelt, & Loprinzi, 2003). Antiseizure medications, such as gabapentin, also have provided symptomatic relief from hot flashes (Loprinzi et al., 2007). NCI (2007) currently is conducting a trial comparing soy and venlafaxine alone or in combination for hot flash management in men receiving ADT for prostate cancer.

Osteoporosis

The patient's susceptibility to bone fractures increases if receiving hormonal manipulation for longer than one year (National Comprehensive Cancer Network [NCCN], 2008c). Baseline and yearly bone density studies should be part of a patient's initial assessment and ongoing management (Otto, 2004). In addition, patients at risk for osteopenia or osteoporosis should perform weight-bearing exercise and receive daily oral supplements of 500 mg of calcium and 400 IU of vitamin D (NCCN, 2008c). Lastly, bisphosphonate therapy, including agents such as zoledronic acid, pamidronate, raloxifene, and toremifene, should be considered in this patient population. Evidence suggests that intermittent use of bisphosphonates in men receiving ADT also prevents osteoporosis (NCCN,

Table 6-1. Side Effect Profiles for Commonly Prescribed Agents Used as Part of Androgen Deprivation Therapy		
Category	Medication Class	Long-Terms Effects
Category A	Luteinizing hormone-releasing hormone agents	Hot flashes, bone pain, peripheral edema, impotence, gynecomastia, fatigue, osteopenia, osteoporosis
Category B	Antiandrogen agents	In addition to those listed in category A: Nausea, headache, fluid retention, weight gain, decreased libido
Category C	Nonsteroidal antiandrogen agents	In addition to those in categories A and B: Diarrhea, nocturia, generalized pain

Note. Based on information from Otto, 2004.

Figure 6-1. Interventions to Assist in Coping With Hot Flashes

- Dress in layers.
- Wear loosely woven cotton or rayon clothes, including at night.
- Use cotton sheets.
- Lower the thermostat, and use air conditioning, a ceiling fan, or a handheld fan.
- Try relaxation exercises, such as deep breathing, guided imagery, hypnosis, biofeedback, and acupuncture.
- Use cold compresses.
- Avoid alcohol, caffeine, and spicy foods, and reduce intake of refined sugar.

Note. Based on information from Fortenbaugh & Rummel, 2007; Polovich et al., 2005.

2008c). A review of the literature on the pathogenesis, diagnosis, prevalence, prevention, and treatment of bone loss in patients with nonmetastatic prostate cancer receiving ADT revealed that the most significant bone mineral density loss occurred within one year of starting ADT and that most fractures occurred in those without osteoporosis. Early intervention is warranted to prevent skeletal morbidity. Most of the evidence supports the use of bisphosphonates, but further research is necessary (Israeli, Ryan, & Jung, 2008).

Erectile Dysfunction

Also known as impotence, erectile dysfunction can occur as a result of radical prostatectomy, RT, or hormonal manipulation. Loss of libido among men undergoing hormonal manipulation is not uncommon. However, many men will still be able to achieve and maintain an erection following ADT (Polovich, White, & Kelleher, 2005). Assessment of sexual dysfunction is extremely important, as it often is underassessed and underaddressed. Oncology nurses should inquire about changes in libido, sleep, mood, erectile function, ability to achieve an orgasm, and gynecomastia (Polovich et al.). For criteria on assessing and grading gynecomastia,

see Table 5-1 in Chapter 5. In addition, assessment should include baseline sexual frequency, quality of the erection, ability to ejaculate, retrograde ejaculation, sensation during intercourse, and satisfaction with intercourse (Shell, 2007). For assessing erectile dysfunction, see Figures 5-5 and 5-6 in Chapter 5. Assessment of sexual issues can be incorporated into the general assessment of treatment-related side effects. Comorbidities such as hypertension, diabetes, peripheral neuropathy, and peripheral vascular disease, all of which have an impact on impotence, should be considered. Review current herbal and nonherbal medications for potential interactions. Inquire as to the presence of stress, recent major lifestyle changes, and impaired coping—all of which may influence erectile dysfunction.

The patient and his partner should verbalize the importance of communication between each other regarding concerns related to sexual dysfunction. The patient should verbalize his understanding of side effects related to sexual dysfunction. Furthermore, the patient and his partner should be made aware of available medical and surgical interventions used to treat sexual dysfunction as well as the side effects associated with these interventions. These interventions are detailed in Chapter 5.

Management of erectile dysfunction has many facets and is a collaborative effort. Most couples do not realize the many possible solutions to restoring sexual intimacy following treatment for prostate cancer. Oncology nurses should encourage discussion regarding this difficult issue and, if necessary, encourage referral to the appropriate healthcare provider for professional counseling. All members of the healthcare team should be sensitive to the difficult nature of this topic and be able to engage in an open and frank discussion about sexual concerns. The patient's urologist should be knowledgeable and skilled in the large variety of surgical and nonsurgical options for restoring sexual function. Some interventions to manage impotence include oral medications such as phosphodiesterase-5 inhibitors, intraurethral suppositories, penile injections, vacuum devices, and penile prostheses.

In one study, men and women both expressed a need for more information upon discharge regarding management of sexual concerns following prostate cancer treatment (Sanders, Pedro, Bantum, & Galbraith, 2006). Information requested included personal experiences and coping mechanisms used by other couples having been through similar treatment. However, in this study, men and women differed in the manner in which they preferred to receive the information. Women desired to participate in support groups with other women present, and men desired to obtain the information through written materials. Oncology nurses should utilize appropriate communication methods to encourage couples dealing with prostate cancer to express their intimacy and communication needs.

Fatigue

Fatigue is a multifactorial, common late effect in cancer survivors. It can occur as a result of any of the treatment modalities for prostate cancer. Fatigue also can result from chronic side effects such as bone pain or bone marrow suppression. Psychosocial distress is another cause of fatigue in many cancer survivors. Several years after treatment, cancer survivors still have increased levels of circulating interleukin-1, tumor necrosis factor, and neopterin, and lower levels of cortisol, all of which validate a biologic basis for long-term fatigue. Patients report distress from experiencing fatigue years following treatment, especially when society expects them to "move on" shortly after treatment is completed. Most patients will experience a gradual decrease in fatigue and a return of normal energy levels. The timing of the return of normal energy levels is individual and can take months after treatment is completed (NCCN, 2008b).

According to NCCN (2008b) guidelines, fatigue is a subjective experience that should be systematically assessed using patient self-reports and other sources of data. Regular self-monitoring of fatigue is helpful in documenting any decreases in fatigue levels that routinely occur after treatment. Fatigue is now known as the sixth vital sign, and as such, patients should be asked to rate fatigue levels. This can be done using a scale of mild, moderate, or severe fatigue or the 0–10 scale, with 0 being equivalent to no fatigue and 10 being equivalent to the worst fatigue imaginable (NCCN,

2008b). Another common fatigue measurement tool is the Functional Assessment of Cancer Therapy–Fatigue (FACT-F) (Cella et al., 1993). The FACT-F utilizes a questionnaire in which patients are asked to rate, using a Likert scale, their perception regarding physical well-being, social and family well-being, emotional well-being, functional well-being, and fatigue. The tool has been proved reliable by test/retest method ($r = .87$ and internal consistency rating of 0.95–0.96 coefficient alpha range). The fatigue subscale was tested as valid via convergent/divergent methodology ($r = .66$) (Yellen, Cella, Webster, Blendowski, & Kaplan, 1997). Of note, the FACT-F is available in 45 different language translations. The NCI CTCAE is helpful when attempting to grade and document a patient's level of fatigue (NCI CTEP, 2006) (see Table 6-2). Educating patients about fatigue begins prior to initiating treatment. Upon completion of treatment, patients and significant others should be informed about the pattern and level of fatigue one can expect during the follow-up period (NCCN, 2008b). If patients expect from the onset that long-term fatigue is a possibility, they may be better prepared to manage it. See Figure 6-2 for fatigue management tips as put forth by NCCN.

Weight Gain

Weight gain is a distressing issue for many men undergoing hormonal manipulation. Basaria et al. (2002) examined weight loss as a long-term effect among men with prostate cancer who had undergone ADT. Patients had received ADT for a range of 12–101 months. When compared to the control group, the ADT group had higher fat mass and significantly reduced upper body strength. Patients experiencing such body changes can be referred to a dietitian or nutritionist for assistance in managing these symptoms. Dietitians also can be helpful in managing other ADT-related side effects, such as nausea and diarrhea. A physical therapy consultation may be useful to devise an exercise program to help men to manage weight gain along with dietary modification. Rehabilitative and nutrition services are increasingly becoming components of oncology survivorship programs (Ganzer & Selle, 2006; Taylor et al., 2006).

Table 6-2. Common Terminology Criteria for Adverse Events for Fatigue						
		Grade				
Adverse Event	Short Name	1	2	3	4	5
Fatigue (asthenia, lethargy, malaise)	Fatigue	Mild fatigue over baseline	Moderate or causing difficulty performing some ADL	Severe fatigue interfering with ADL	Disabling	–

ADL—activities of daily living

Note. From *Common Terminology Criteria for Adverse Events* (Version 3.0, p. 11), by National Cancer Institute Cancer Therapy Evaluation Program, 2006. Retrieved March 14, 2008, from http://ctep.cancer.gov/forms/CTCAEv3.pdf

---

Figure 6-2. Fatigue Management Tips for Survivors of Prostate Cancer

- Make a list of activities that you need to do, and rate their importance. Plan to do the high-priority items at a time when you have the most energy.
- Ask for help and delegate tasks whenever possible. When people ask what they can do for you, give them a task.
- Establish a daily routine.
- Keep a fatigue journal. Note when you feel you are most fatigued and least fatigued.
- Use methods to reduce stress, such as deep breathing, guided imagery, meditation, prayer, and activities that give you pleasure.
- If you are experiencing pain, anxiety, or depression, talk with your doctor about how to manage these symptoms.
- Minimize extended napping during the day. Shorter rest periods are reported to be better than longer ones.
- Get fresh air if possible.
- Balance rest and physical activities.
- Maintain physical activities as normally as possible.
- Eat a balanced diet, and drink at least 8–10 glasses of water a day.

Note. Based on information from National Comprehensive Cancer Network, 2008b.

Chemotherapy

Little is known about the long-term effects of chemotherapy in patients with prostate cancer, as chemotherapy historically has shown little benefit. Chemotherapeutic agents, when prescribed for this patient population, mainly are used with palliative intent. Patients with advanced prostate cancer eventually become refractory to hormonal manipulation, thereby leaving chemotherapy as an end-stage option. According to NCCN (2008c), systemic chemotherapy with a docetaxel-based regimen should be reserved for patients with castration-recurrent (surgical or medical) metastatic prostate cancer. When managing survivorship issues in patients with advanced prostate cancer who have received chemotherapy, nurses must assess for late side effects as the patient's life span permits. Active combination agents often administered at some point in the disease trajectory include docetaxel and prednisone, mitoxantrone and prednisone, and docetaxel and estramustine. Patients with rapidly progressing soft-tissue disease or those who have visceral or lytic bone lesions and a low PSA level are managed with cisplatin and etoposide or carboplatin and etoposide (NCCN, 2008c).

Chemotherapy affects virtually every organ in the body, and long-term effects vary among patients. Therefore, assessment of long-term effects should take place during each follow-up visit. Chemotherapy can cause annoying and sometimes debilitating long-term effects, such as neurotoxicity (ototoxicity, peripheral neuropathy), fluid retention, and bone marrow suppression, especially if given to a patient who may have received RT.

Neurotoxicity

Neurotoxicity affects almost half of patients with all types of cancers receiving docetaxel (Wilkes & Barton-Burke, 2007). This number is higher in patients receiving concurrent cisplatin or for those who have preexisting neuropathy from other comorbidities. In a study evaluating docetaxel versus mitoxantrone for treatment of metastatic prostate cancer, 30% of patients developed sensory neuropathy in the every-three-week docetaxel arm, versus 24% in the weekly docetaxel arm, versus 7% in the mitoxantrone alone every-three-week arm (Tannock et al., 2004). In another study, 21% of men with metastatic prostate cancer receiving docetaxel and estramustine experienced grade 3 neurologic adverse events and 2% experienced grade 4 neurologic events, as compared with a similarly matched group of men receiving mitoxantrone and prednisone, in which 5% experienced grade 3 neurologic events and no men experienced grade 4 events (Petrylak et al., 2004).

Assessment of baseline neurologic motor and sensory function prior to chemotherapy administration is important. The presence and severity of numbness and tingling in the hands or feet should be addressed. The presence or absence of pain is not necessarily indicative of neuropathy, as patients may not perceive numbness and tingling as pain. Techniques used to assess peripheral neuropathy may include the patient's ability to pick up a coin from a flat surface or unbutton/button clothing. Further assessment for a "stocking-glove distribution" of neuropathy should take place. Stocking-glove distribution describes neuropathy as beginning in the fingertips or toes and moving in a proximal direction as when one dons a stocking or glove. In addition, careful assessment of the patient's ability to sense changes in temperature is important, as is assessment of sensory changes when walking. Consideration should be given to withholding or dose-reducing chemotherapy if neurotoxicity reaches grade 3 as measured by the CTCAE toxicity scale (NCI, 2006). For criteria to determine the degree of sensory or motor neuropathy according to the CTCAE, see Table 6-3.

Although chemotherapy-induced peripheral neuropathy typically is seen in the hands or feet, patients should be encouraged to report any sensory changes or numbness from anywhere within the body. When neuropathy is present, the patient should be informed of safety measures such as removing area rugs, adjusting hot water temperature, protecting extremities from extreme temperatures, and placing handrails in the bathroom or near staircases as necessary (Wilkes & Barton-Burke, 2007). Neurotoxicity is medically managed by a variety of agents, including the anticonvulsant gabapentin, short- and long-acting opioids, SSRIs and norepinephrine inhibitors, systemic and local anesthetic agents such as a lidocaine patch 5%, topical capsaicin, and tricyclic antidepressants, such as amitriptyline. Nonpharmacologic management includes exercise, massage, imagery, hypnosis, and hydrotherapy (NCCN, 2008a), as well as acupuncture

Table 6-3. Common Terminology Criteria for Adverse Events (Version 3.0) for Sensory and Motor Neuropathy

Adverse Event	Short Name	Grade				
		1	2	3	4	5
Neuropathy: motor	Neuropathy-motor	Asymptomatic, weakness on exam/testing only	Symptomatic weakness interfering with function, but not interfering with ADL	Weakness interfering with ADL; bracing or assistance to walk (e.g., cane or walker) indicated	Life-threatening; disabling	Death
Remark: Cranial nerve <u>motor</u> neuropathy is graded as Neuropathy: cranial – *Select*. Also Consider: Laryngeal nerve dysfunction; Phrenic nerve dysfunction.						
Neuropathy: sensory	Neuropathy-sensory	Asymptomatic; loss of deep tendon reflexes or paresthesia (including tingling) but not interfering with function	Sensory alteration or paresthesia (including tingling), interfering with function, but not interfering with ADL	Sensory alteration or paresthesia interfering with ADL	Disabling	Death
Remark: Cranial nerve <u>sensory</u> neuropathy is graded as Neuropathy: cranial – *Select*.						

ADL—activities of daily living

Note. From *Common Terminology Criteria for Adverse Events* (Version 3.0, p. 50), by National Cancer Institute Cancer Therapy Evaluation Program, 2006. Retrieved March 14, 2008, from http://ctep.cancer.gov/forms/CTCAEv3.pdf

and magnet therapy (Abuaisha, Costanzi, & Boulton, 1998; Weintraub et al., 2003). Brunelli and Gorson (2004) surveyed 180 outpatients with peripheral neuropathy, of which 77 (43%) respondents reported using complementary and alternative medicine. The most frequent interventions reported were megavitamins (35%), magnets (30%), acupuncture (30%), herbal remedies (22%), and chiropractic manipulation (21%). Also, 48% of the respondents admitted to using more than one form of alternative treatment.

Physical or occupational therapists should be included in the collaborative management of patients with peripheral neuropathy for strengthening exercises and for assistance with any devices that may help in adaptive functioning (Armstrong, Almadrones, & Gilbert, 2005).

Ototoxicity

A form of autonomic neurotoxicity, ototoxicity affects almost 30% of patients receiving cisplatin (Wilkes & Barton-Burke, 2007). Patients receiving cisplatin should have a baseline audiogram (Armstrong et al., 2005), and it should be repeated prior to each subsequent dose so that if ototoxicity occurs, its extent can be detected and measured (Bedford Laboratories, 2004). Ototoxicity has been observed in up to 31% of patients treated with a single dose of cisplatin of 50 mg/m². It is manifested by tinnitus or hearing loss in the high-frequency range of 4,000–8,000 hertz. Ability to hear normal conversational tones also may decrease. Hearing loss can be

either unilateral or bilateral and becomes more frequent and severe with repeated doses of cisplatin. It may become more severe in patients being treated with other drugs that have nephrotoxic potential (Bedford Laboratories).

Fluid Retention

Fluid retention is a cumulative toxicity in patients receiving docetaxel and usually resolves within 16 weeks of the last dose (Wilkes & Barton-Burke, 2007). The range of time during which fluid retention may persist is 0–42 weeks following the completion of treatment (Wilkes & Barton-Burke). Fluid retention may cause patients to experience generalized edema, peripheral edema, pleural effusion, dyspnea at rest, cardiac tamponade, or ascites. Assessment of fluid retention should include monitoring the patient's weight, skin integrity and turgor, presence or absence of edema (especially in the extremities), respiratory pattern, breath sounds, coughing, abdominal girth, sense of bloating, and excessive belching or hiccups as a result of diaphragm displacement from excessive fluid.

Patients should be instructed to report any new onset of the previously listed symptoms. Patients with fluid retention usually are asked to restrict sodium intake, and a dietary consult may be helpful in this regard. Management of fluid retention starts proactively, and the administration of oral dexamethasone 8 mg BID for three days prior to initiating chemotherapy may help in minimizing one's overall volume of fluid retention. Diuretics also may be prescribed for new onset of edema, progression of edema, or a weight gain of more than two pounds (Wilkes & Barton-Burke, 2007).

Bone Marrow Suppression

Patients who have received RT to the pelvis and systemic chemotherapy at some point during the disease trajectory should be monitored for hematologic toxicity. Thus, blood counts should be monitored on a regular basis. When administered independently of one another, chemotherapy and RT used to treat prostate cancer are unlikely to cause significant pancytopenia. However, when given sequentially, some patients may be more likely to have long-term bone marrow suppression as evidenced by decreased blood counts. Additionally, if advanced metastatic prostate cancer is present, a mild to moderate degree of anemia may persist, as a significant portion of stem cell–producing bone marrow may be replaced by active tumor.

Radiation Therapy

Late effects of RT for prostate cancer, whether external beam or brachytherapy, can occur months to years following treatment. Such effects are a result of damage to the microcirculation and neurogenic pathways of the urinary bladder, rectum, and penis, the severity of which depends on the dose of radiation. The higher the dose per fraction, the more severe the late effects will likely be. Standard radiation doses for low-risk disease patients are 70–75 gray (Gy) (NCCN, 2008c) in 35–41 fractions to the prostate with or without radiation to the seminal vesicles. Moderate- and high-risk patients are offered external beam radiation with either short-term (six months) or long-term (two years) androgen deprivation. Patient selection is dependent on Gleason score and PSA level. Radiation doses for this subset of patients range from 75–80 Gy (NCCN, 2008c). Typical dose per fraction ranges from 1.8–2 Gy. The presence of early side effects does not accurately predict the incidence and degree of late effects. The extent of tissue injury from radiation varies from patient to patient. Follow-up care should be coordinated among the radiation oncologist, urologist, and medical oncologist. Late effects that may result from RT used to definitively treat prostate cancer include chronic gastrointestinal (GI) changes, particularly diarrhea, which in turn affects the patient's nutritional status; urinary symptoms such as dysuria, frequency, and incontinence; and erectile dysfunction.

Gastrointestinal

Irradiation to the lower abdomen and pelvis causes vascular insufficiency as well as damage to surrounding connective tissue. Radiation to healthy digestive tissue can cause chronic changes in normal physiologic function, which ultimately has an adverse impact on the digestion and absorption of nutrients. The volume of the bowel in the treatment field affects the incidence and type of complications. Chronic digestive toxicity includes diarrhea, maldigestion, malabsorption, chronic colitis and enteritis, ulceration, stricture, chronic bleeding, abscess and fistula formation, obstruction, and perforation. These chronic symptoms may not appear for months or years after treatment. Median onset for symptoms to develop is 8–12 months but can occur up to 15 years following radiation (Bruner, Haas, & Gosselin-Acomb, 2005). Of patients receiving radiation to the lower abdomen and pelvis, 5%–15% experience chronic effects (Bruner et al.). Late rectal symptoms related to RT include tenesmus, fecal urge, and fecal incontinence. These symptoms occur in a minority of patients and intermittently, usually less than once a week (Bruner et al.). Geinitz et al. (2006) reported a high correlation between late bowel dysfunction, particularly diarrhea and fecal incontinence, and QOL. Researchers looked at the prevalence of late rectal symptoms and QOL in patients who received conformal RT for localized prostate cancer. A total of 249 patients were interviewed 24–111 months after therapy. The median dose of radiation received was 70 Gy. QOL was assessed using the European Organisation for Research and Treatment of Cancer Quality of Life Questionnaire C30 and the Prostate Cancer Module (PR25). The study showed that both rectal symptoms and fecal incontinence were intermittent. Daily symptoms occurred in 5% of patients or less. Fecal incontinence, fecal urge, and tenesmus were associated with lower global QOL levels. This study underscored that late treatment side effects do affect QOL, and patients must be aware of these factors when making treatment decisions (Nandipati, Raina, Agarwal, & Zippe, 2007).

The incidence of GI and urinary side effects is lower with intensity-modulated radiation therapy (IMRT) when compared to standard external beam or three-dimensional RT to the prostate gland (Ashman, Zelefsky, Hunt, Leibel, & Fuks, 2005; DeMeerleer et al., 2007; Shu et al., 2001; Zelefsky et al., 1999, 2002). IMRT is a more advanced RT technique that allows for the variation of radiation dose to a target, in this case the prostate, and surrounding tissue, thus further decreasing toxicity to the bladder, small bowel, and rectum while allowing for dose escalation. The intensity of the beam is modulated intentionally, allowing for therapeutic radiation doses of 70–80 Gy (NCCN, 2008c). IMRT is replacing three-dimensional conformal RT as the standard of care for prostate cancer at most major cancer centers (Hogle, 2007).

When assessing for late GI-related toxicity from radiation, the following should be considered: prior abdominal surgery, total dose of radiation to the bowel, presence of pelvic inflammatory diseases, colitis, and comorbidities affecting blood flow, such as diabetes, cardiovascular disease, and hypertension (Bruner et al., 2005). Assessment parameters should include the patient's general appearance, height, weight, body mass index, and nutritional status, including daily intake of fluids, calories, and protein. The patient may need to keep a food diary to gauge current intake. Review usual elimination patterns, and note any changes. If diarrhea is present, note the onset, frequency, amount, and character of stool as well as the presence of blood in the stool. Note the presence or absence of symptoms suggestive of dehydration such as poor skin turgor, dry mucous membranes, and elevated serum blood urea nitrogen level with normal creatinine. The scored Patient-Generated Subjective Global Assessment (PG-SGA) tool is a validated, reliable assessment measure for the standardized nutritional care of patients with cancer. This assessment tool is accepted as the standard by the American Dietetic Association (ADA). The PG-SGA was developed specifically for use in patients with cancer. It allows quick identification and prioritization of nutritional deficiencies in patients. The PG-SGA score is correlated with objective parameters, such as percentage weight loss, body mass index, and measures of morbidity, and it has a high degree of inter-rater reproducibility when compared with other validated nutritional assessment tools. This tool has a section for the patient to complete and a section for the healthcare provider to complete (Ottery, 2000).

Other factors to consider include the patients' perceived level of stress, coping patterns, and impact of symptoms on their usual lifestyle. Lastly, concurrent medications, including any over-the-counter or herbal supplements, should be evaluated for possible GI-related distress.

Patients should be instructed to report any signs or symptoms of late GI effects, such as diarrhea, rectal pain, or rectal bleeding. Reinforce the importance of long-term follow-up. If diarrhea occurs, instruct the patient to record the number and consistency of bowel movements. Avoiding consumption of fried foods or foods high in fat, milk-based food products, foods high in fiber such as raw fruits and vegetables, large amounts of fruit juice and sweetened fruit drinks, cereals, whole-grain breads, seeds, skins, spicy foods, caffeine, alcohol, and tobacco is helpful in reducing the severity of diarrhea (Bruner et al., 2005). A low-residue diet, such as baked, boiled, or steamed meat, poultry or fish, refined grains, cooked vegetables, canned fruit, applesauce, bananas, and juices and nectars, is recommended (Bruner et al.). Instruct patients about skin care and incontinence products if applicable. Lastly, patients should be informed of the signs and symptoms of dehydration, such as excessive thirst, fever, dizziness, light-headedness, headache, and palpitations.

Treatment of late GI toxicity, in terms of medical management, is similar to treatment given for acute distress. Chronic rectal bleeding may be treated with long-term steroid application, laser therapy, fulguration (a procedure to destroy tissue using an electric current), or formalin instillation. If a partial bowel obstruction occurs, it may resolve without surgical intervention. A complete bowel obstruction, be it mechanical in nature or from scarring or fibrosis, frequently requires surgical intervention. When chronic GI symptoms are present, it is best to include a gastroenterologist and general surgeon in the patient's management.

Coping with chronic GI toxicities can be life altering. Although cure is always paramount, practitioners sometimes fail to fully realize that long-term effects from treatment can significantly alter one's QOL and serve as a constant reminder of malignancy. Dietary modifications, personal hygiene, and long-term use of medications can be an emotional and financial burden. Emotional support for patients and loved ones should be encouraged, and nurses who are skilled in this practice should intervene as appropriate. Additionally, a consult to behavioral medicine should be considered. See Table 6-4 for dietary resources available to survivors of prostate cancer.

Genitourinary

The most common late genitourinary effects from radiation to the prostate include dysuria, urinary incontinence, and erectile dysfunction. The effects of radiation on the urothelial lining include edema, irritation, inflammation, and vascular changes of the urinary bladder and smooth muscle. The exact mechanism that causes urinary incontinence in this setting is not well known. It may be caused by tissue damage and decreased urethral closing related to dry, thin fibrosed tissue. Radiation-induced cystitis can occur, although this rarely

Table 6-4. Dietary Resources for Prostate Cancer Survivors	
Resource	Web Site
A Dietitian's Cancer Story	www.cancerrd.com
American Dietetic Association	www.eatright.org
American Cancer Society: Nutrition After Treatment Ends	www.cancer.org/docroot/MBC/content/MBC_6_2X_Nutrition_after_treatment_ends.asp
American Institute for Cancer Research	www.aicr.org (Contains recipes and information for cancer prevention and survivorship)
Note. Based on information from Bruner et al., 2005.	

lasts more than three to five weeks following the completion of therapy. Tissue damage related to interstitial fibrosis results in thin-walled bladder vessels, which can rupture, thus resulting in painless hematuria. Irradiated epithelial tissue becomes thin, pale, and atrophied and may ulcerate (Bruner et al., 2005; Hogle, 2007).

Assessment of late urinary effects includes inquiring about the presence of urinary burning, urgency, frequency, dysuria, hematuria, and nocturia. Urinary bladder distention or tenderness of the bladder upon palpation may indicate urinary retention, cystitis, or possible infection. Presence of fever or a positive urine culture is a strong indicator of a urinary tract infection. Determining a patient's American Urological Association (AUA) score upon initial evaluation and during subsequent follow-up appointments may be helpful, along with follow-up exams after intervention. The present AUA scoring system is derived from an index of seven questions to which patients respond by providing answers in the form of a numeric value (Nitti, Kim, & Combs, 1994). When AUA scoring is used, the total score is classified as mild (0–7), moderate (8–19), or severe (20–35). Originally derived from a more extensive survey to determine the degree of bothersome urinary symptoms experienced by patients with benign prostatic hypertrophy, the AUA index has demonstrated high internal consistency (Cronbach's alpha = 0.86) and high test-retest reliability (r = .92) (Barry et al., 1992). It is believed that patients with a higher pretreatment AUA score may have a higher degree of urinary morbidity secondary to radiation.

Late urinary effects generally are managed by long-term administration of urinary analgesics, antispasmodics, and alpha-1 receptor blocking agents. These same agents are used to treat acute urinary distress from RT. Please see Chapter 5 for a review of these agents along with appropriate administration schedules. When patients are on long-term use of any medication, oncology practitioners should continue to assess for and educate patients about potential side effects. In addition, possible interactions with other medications, including herbals and drug/food interactions, should be reviewed and

is an important part of ongoing medication reconciliation. If decreased bladder capacity or urinary outlet obstruction continues, endoscopic examination and possible urethral dilation may be indicated. In addition to medication administration, patients should be encouraged to eliminate caffeinated beverages from their diet and to drink one to two liters of fluid during daytime hours to reduce the incidence of nocturia (Hogle, 2007).

Assessment and interventions for incontinence are discussed in more detail in the surgery section of this chapter and in Chapter 5 of this text. See Table 6-5 for criteria to evaluate the degree of urinary incontinence as determined by the CTCAE (NCI CTEP, 2006).

Erectile Dysfunction

Another chronic late effect of radiation to the prostate gland is erectile dysfunction. It generally occurs six to eight months after the completion of treatment and is the result of a disruption of the arteriolar system that supplies the corporal muscles of the penis. The incidence of erectile dysfunction varies greatly, 6%–84% according to Incrocci, Slob, and Levendag (2002), and is believed to be influenced significantly by the size of the treatment field, age of the patient, and the presence of comorbid conditions. It is not uncommon for most men who have undergone radiation treatments for prostate cancer to experience some degree of erectile dysfunction at some point during their remaining life. Some data suggest that treatment using IMRT may result in improved potency rates (Brown, Brooks, Albert, & Poggi, 2007); however, additional studies are needed to confirm this, especially when compared to traditional external beam or three-dimensional RT. Radiation also can affect ejaculatory function, including a reduction or absence of ejaculate, hematospermia, or painful ejaculation.

Assessment of erectile dysfunction should include inquiry as to the presence and firmness of erections and the ability to achieve vaginal penetration adequate for orgasm and mutual

Table 6-5. Common Terminology Criteria for Adverse Events (Version 3.0) for Urinary Incontinence

Adverse Event	Short Name	Grade 1	2	3	4	5
Incontinence, urinary	Incontinence, urinary	Occasional (e.g., with coughing, sneezing, etc.), pads not indicated	Spontaneous, pads indicated	Interfering with ADL; intervention indicated (e.g., clamp, collagen injections)	Operative intervention indicated (e.g., cystectomy or permanent urinary diversion)	–

ADL—activities of daily living

Note. From *Common Terminology Criteria for Adverse Events* (Version 3.0, p. 60), by National Cancer Institute Cancer Therapy Evaluation Program, 2006. Retrieved March 14, 2008, from http://ctep.cancer.gov/forms/CTCAEv3.pdf

sexual satisfaction. Other considerations include one's libido, degree of satisfaction with one's own sex life, and presence of an interested partner.

Management of erectile dysfunction involves a collaborative approach. Medical intervention has been covered in the hormonal therapy section of this chapter and in greater detail in Chapter 5. The long-term effects of erectile dysfunction can be problematic to survivors of prostate cancer and their sexual partners. The importance of professional counseling regarding the physical and psychological effects of any degree of sexual dysfunction in cancer survivors should not be overlooked (Bruner et al., 2005). Nurses should encourage support groups and ongoing behavioral or sex therapy.

Surgery

Because most men who are surgical candidates are expected to survive for a lengthy period of time, care must be taken upon diagnosis to select the surgical procedure and treatment plan that is associated with the greatest survival benefit and the least long-term side effects. Oncology nurses working with this patient population have the opportunity to help men to understand survivorship issues upon diagnosis. Candidates for radical prostatectomy must be in good physical condition, 70 years old or younger, with a life expectancy of 10–20 years (NCCN, 2008c). In general, men who undergo radical prostatectomy report more urinary side effects and sexual dysfunction and improved bowel function when compared to men who had undergone radiation for definitive treatment (Blank & Bellizzi, 2006). Prostatectomy without the use of a nerve-sparing technique causes a high rate of long-term incontinence and impotence following the procedure (NCCN, 2007). The more nerve pathways spared, the lower the incidence of incontinence and impotence. In addition, bladder neck contracture may result following radical prostatectomy.

Minimally invasive prostatectomy techniques are covered in Chapter 4. In general, these techniques utilize smaller incisions and smaller instrumentation, which tends to result in decreased rates of incontinence and impotence compared to traditional surgery (Tewari et al., 2002). However, a steep learning curve exists for physicians who perform minimally invasive prostatectomy. Thus, they should be performed at a facility where a high volume of cases are performed on a yearly basis. In one descriptive study, 66% of 212 men who had undergone radical prostatectomy at least one year prior reported decreased urinary function, and 36.3% reported that bowel habits were problematic. Furthermore, these symptoms had affected the participants' overall QOL. Additionally, 41% of respondents stated upon discharge that they were not informed about the possibility of urinary incontinence and sexual problems following prostate surgery (O'Connel, Baker, & Munro, 2007), thus suggesting a need for additional information about side effects and potential complications of treatment. Oncology nurses have the responsibility of providing information to patients about the possibility of late urinary incontinence and impotence during the perioperative period.

In another study, researchers assessed incontinence rates in 152 men who underwent radical prostatectomy with nerve sparing on one side, both sides, or with no attempt at nerve sparing (Nandipati et al., 2007). During these surgeries, it often is difficult not to injure the nerves surrounding the prostate. After an average follow-up period of 7.8 years, 27 patients (17.7%) experienced urinary incontinence. Eighteen of the 61 patients treated with non-nerve-sparing surgery were incontinent, compared with just 6 of the 66 men who underwent nerve-sparing surgery on both sides—a statistically significant difference. However, the surgical approach that only partially preserved the nerves offered no benefits over surgery that did not spare the nerves at all. In addition to the type of surgery, patient age also affected incontinence rates. Men who were older than 65 years were significantly more likely to become incontinent than were younger patients. These findings suggested that, whenever medically feasible, all men may benefit from nerve-sparing prostate surgery. The radical form of the surgery, usually performed in men with prostate cancer as opposed to those with noncancerous prostate disease, involves the complete removal of the gland.

When assessing urinary incontinence, nurses should consider the type and extent of prostate surgery performed. Also, the nurse should determine the length of time that has passed since surgery because, in most cases, incontinence gradually diminishes (O'Rourke, 2005). The type of incontinence from which the patient suffers—stress, overflow, or urge (see Table 5-6)—also is important. Stress incontinence, the most common type of incontinence following prostatectomy, typically is treated with surgery. Severe incontinence may require urinary diversion (ileal conduit) (Ahmed & Davies, 2005). Patients with persistent incontinence should be referred to a wound, ostomy, and continence nurse for consultation. The overall effectiveness of conservative management of postprostatectomy urinary incontinence remains unclear, and further phase III trials are needed to fully evaluate current interventions (Hunter, Moore, & Glazener, 2007). Detailed management of incontinence is described in great detail in Chapter 5. The emotional and financial issues facing men with urinary incontinence are similar to those who experience bowel incontinence. Oncology nurses should provide emotional support and information as to the availability of support groups and financial resources within the community. Behavioral medicine may be necessary to include as part of the collaborative team, as long-term incontinence potentially may cause feelings of isolation, embarrassment, anger, and resentment.

Psychosocial Issues

Psychosocial issues in survivors of prostate cancer encompass the whole being: mind, body, and spirit. In general, cancer survivors raise psychosocial concerns related to at least one of the following issues: sexual dysfunction, employment, fear and anxiety regarding cancer recurrence, body image, changes in degree of social interaction, questioning treatment decision (e.g., Did I do the right thing?), altered roles and relationships, and depression.

Most men cope well with being long-term survivors of prostate cancer. Some evidence has shown that well-being and adaptive lifestyle changes after a diagnosis of prostate cancer are affected by the patient's personality factors, coping strategies, primary treatment, and stage upon diagnosis. Men who report more negative outcomes, such as depression, are likely to be those who continue to be affected by the disease years after treatment and thereby continue to engage in a range of coping strategies (Blank & Bellizzi, 2006). Nurses should not underestimate patients' desire for knowledge regarding their disease state. One study of prostate cancer survivors reported that patients who did not receive the desired amount of information about psychosocial implications of treatment reported a significantly higher level of stress than their counterparts who perceived that enough information about psychosocial implications had been provided (Hyacinth, Thibault, & Ruttle-King, 2006).

Personal Distress

The NCCN distress guidelines provide an excellent starting point from which oncology nurses can assess psychosocial issues in prostate cancer survivors. NCCN (2007) defined distress as a multifactorial, unpleasant emotional experience of a psychological (cognitive, behavioral, emotional), social, or spiritual nature that may interfere with one's ability to cope effectively with cancer, its physical symptoms, and its treatment. Distress extends along a continuum, ranging from common normal feelings of vulnerability, sadness, and fear about the future, to problems that can be disabling, such as depression, anxiety, panic, social isolation, and existential and spiritual crisis. The NCCN panel chose the word *distress* to characterize the psychosocial aspects of patient care because it is less stigmatizing and more acceptable than other terms (NCCN, 2007).

The first section of the validated NCCN distress measurement screening tool is called the distress thermometer, which requires the patient to rate on a scale of 0–10 that which best describes the amount of distress experienced within the past week. Zero is equivalent to no distress, and 10 is equivalent to extreme distress. A score less than four indicates a normal response to cancer diagnosis and treatment, and the oncology team may choose to handle the problem or recommend a support group. A score of four or higher indicates a significant level of distress that should be further evaluated. The nurse, social worker, or oncologist determines whether the patient has significant distress. The problem list, which is on the same page as the distress thermometer in the NCCN

(2007) guidelines, asks the patient to identify problems such as those that are physical (including appearance, bathing and dressing, memory, and concentration), practical (such as transportation), psychological, social, or spiritual. Patients can do so by indicating a *yes* or *no* response as to whether they have experienced problems or concerns during the past week. NCCN recommends that patients complete the distress-screening tool in the physician's waiting room prior to their appointment time. Patients need to understand the importance of reporting their distress and the distress experienced by significant others to the healthcare team. Oncology nurses are central to the assessment of psychosocial issues by their presence throughout all patient visits, their concern for the total patient, their opportunity to ask further questions, and their ability to collaborate with other appropriate members of the healthcare team (NCCN, 2007).

Patients experiencing distress should be referred, as needed, to other collaborative disciplines, such as social workers, pastoral counselors, and behavioral medicine. The goal of distress management is to have a process in place for identifying patients who might benefit from early intervention and referral to appropriate members of the healthcare team (NCCN, 2007).

Sexual Dysfunction

Psychosocial late effects related to sexual dysfunction include poor or distorted self-image, changes in appearance, concerns about attractiveness to partner or feelings toward the partner, difficulties with relationships, concerns about reproductive capacity, social isolation, anxiety, and depression (Polovich et al., 2005). Nurses can use the PLISSIT model when assessing and discussing sexual function. It consists of four stages of intervention. The first stage involves *permission* to ask about sexual concerns. This normalizes the experience and allows patients to discuss their concerns. The next stage involves providing *limited information* while clarifying concerns and misconceptions. Third, the nurse provides *specific suggestions* based on patients' concerns. The last stage is *intensive therapy*. If the first three steps are not helpful, a referral to a sex therapist should be considered (Polovich et al.). Despite the findings that sexuality continues throughout all phases of life, little material—scientific or otherwise—exists in the literature to guide nurses toward assessing the sexuality of older adults. Consequently, validity and reliability evidence to support the PLISSIT model or the suggested questions is not available. Further research in the area of sexuality among older adults is imperative.

Oncology nurses should support patients who have concerns regarding sexual function. Patients should be encouraged to communicate with their partners about fears related to continued sexual function. Lastly, patients should be assured that referrals can be made to a licensed psychologist, clinical social worker, or sex therapist should psychosocial problems regarding sexual dysfunction continue (Bruner et al., 2005).

Fear of Recurrence

Fear and anxiety about cancer recurrence is a common concern for cancer survivors. The healthcare team can make a difference in the long-term psychological well-being of survivors by providing factual information during the decision-making process and by providing long-term support. The healthcare team must realize that long-term support will be necessary (Clark & Talcott, 2006). Men who choose active surveillance are spared acute and late side effects of treatment but may experience increased overall stress and anxiety about the future of their cancer and may experience decreased sexual function. One study also reported that men undergoing surveillance who actively managed their health by altering lifestyle behaviors associated with prostate cancer actually improved their QOL and sexual function, suggesting that the healthier the lifestyle, the better the QOL. Oncology nurses should encourage men receiving active surveillance to partner with their primary care physician to make positive lifestyle changes (Daubenmier et al., 2005). One study examined the impact of comorbidities at diagnosis, post-treatment symptom changes, fear of cancer recurrence, and physical symptoms on both disease-specific QOL and general health-related QOL. Respondents included 1,100 men with localized disease who were identified from a national observational prostate registry. The study showed that new symptoms occurring after treatment affected disease-specific QOL more than fear of recurrence, but both factors were important contributors to general health-related QOL after prostate cancer treatment (Bellizzi, Latini, Cowan, DuChane, & Carroll, 2006).

Outreach and Support

Support groups are one avenue for patients and significant others to discuss and deal with the psychosocial late effects of treatment and, in some cases, physical effects. Nurses can help to educate patients and their families about available support groups in the area, online resources, and organizations designed to assist prostate cancer survivors. Owen, Goldstein, Lee, Breen, and Rowland (2007) reported that oncologists passively supported patient participation in support groups, but only 1 in 10 patients with cancer reported having received a physician recommendation to attend a support group. Assistance in identifying support groups and resources should be the standard of care. See Table 6-6 for a list of available support groups and contact information for prostate cancer survivors.

Workplace Concerns

Prostate cancer survivors may have concerns about employment issues, returning to work and health insurance, and their legal rights once treatment is completed. Several laws exist that protect patients regarding health insurance and related

matters. The Family and Medical Leave Act (FMLA) allows eligible individuals to take up to 12 weeks of unpaid leave beyond sick time, during which an employee can be off from work without penalty. Survivors may already be aware of the FMLA, but this is useful information for those who are worried about job loss resulting from recurrence of their disease. The Consolidated Omnibus Budget Reconciliation Act allows workers the right to continue group health insurance benefits for up to 18 months after job loss occurs. The Health Insurance Portability and Accountability Act prohibits discrimination against employees and their dependents enrolled in group health plans based on their health status and provides for health coverage under group health plans that limit exclusions for preexisting conditions. More information can be obtained about all three pieces of legislation from the U.S. Department of Labor Web site (www.dol.gov). The Americans with Disabilities Act prohibits employment discrimination against qualified individuals with disabilities. More information can be obtained from the U.S. Equal Employment Opportunity Commission's Web site (www.eeoc.gov). The Cancer Survival Toolbox® from NCCS, done in collaboration with the Oncology Nursing Society, is a free audio program designed to help cancer survivors and caregivers to develop practical skills to deal with the diagnosis, treatment, and challenges of cancer. One section of the toolbox has information for patients about employment issues. The toolbox can be ordered from the NCCS Web site (www.cancersurvivaltoolbox.org) or by telephone (877-TOOLS-4U).

Quality of Life

As survival rates for prostate cancer have risen, so too has the focus on survivor QOL. When considering treatment, the potential cure for the disease must be carefully weighed along with the potential impact on QOL. In fact, all prostate cancer treatments carry the risk of side effects that compromise QOL (Albaugh & Hacker, 2008). Much research has been conducted on QOL of patients with cancer. However, only within the past two decades have researchers begun to examine the concept of QOL in patients with prostate cancer. Although a number of definitions for QOL exist in the literature, the general agreement is that it is a multidimensional concept that is individually experienced and includes both positive and negative aspects of one's life. QOL typically encompasses one's physical, psychological, social, economic, and spiritual world. It is a self-perceived notion that is not at all static. It can change often, and numerous factors influence it. Because QOL is such a multidimensional construct, measuring and reporting on QOL indicators can be difficult. Determining which dimensions are most important to men with prostate cancer, and whether they should be measured equally, may provide keen insight and be beneficial to understanding QOL issues (Albaugh & Hacker). QOL measures are important, as

Table 6-6. Resources and Contacts for Prostate Cancer Survivors		
Organization	**Contact Information**	**Description**
American Cancer Society	800-227-2345 www.cancer.org	Offers resources for family and patient support and advocacy as well as research and education
American Urological Association Foundation	866-746-4282 www.auafoundation.org	Advocates for urologic disease research, prevention, education, treatment, and cure
Cancer*Care*	800-813-HOPE www.cancercare.org	Provides support services to patients and families
Lance Armstrong Foundation	866-467-7205 www.livestrong.org	Provides patients with resources for improved quality of life and financial and insurance issues
National Cancer Institute	800-4-CANCER www.cancer.gov	Provides specialists that patients and families can speak to for answers
National Coalition for Cancer Survivorship	877-622-7937 www.canceradvocacy.org	Advocates for cancer care issues at the federal level
National Prostate Cancer Coalition	888-245-9455 www.fightprostatecancer.org	Offers education and free screening and advocates for more research funding
Oncology Nursing Society	866-257-4667 www.cancersymptoms.org	Provides information on education and management of specific cancer-related symptoms
Prostate Cancer Education Council	866-477-6788 www.pcaw.com	Provides information on treatment options
The Prostate Net	888-477-6763 http://prostate-online.org	Provides risk awareness, early detection, and treatment information and support; works with other organizations
Us TOO International Prostate Cancer Education and Support Network	800-808-7866 www.ustoo.org	Provides education through publications and support groups
Wellness Community	888-793-9355 www.thewellnesscommunity.org	Offers support groups, workshops, and programs led by professionals

they provide valuable information about what a patient experiences and how to support and address future needs (Ferrell, Dow, & Grant, 1995; King, 2006).

A number of QOL measurement tools exist in the literature, some of which examine physical well-being (urinary morbidity, urinary incontinence, bowel dysfunction), psychological well-being, social well-being (sexual dysfunction), and spiritual well-being (see Figure 6-3). Some tools are specific to acute side effects, whereas others focus on issues related to chronic or advanced disease. Because so many tools are available, and because so many side effects from treatment affect numerous aspects of one's life, controversy exists as to which tool or tools are most appropriate for use in patients with prostate cancer. In most cases, it might be wise to use a tool that examines issues related to cancer in general and then delves deeper into a specific side effect. Through this approach, researchers are able to obtain both general and specific data sets. Other concerns when using a QOL tool include the use of qualitative or quantitative measures; use of a one-dimensional or multidimensional tool; use of a generic

or cancer-specific tool; and use of single or repeated measures (King, 2006). When deciding on an appropriate measurement tool, it is of utmost importance to use a tool that has been tested and deemed reliable and valid.

Regardless of methodology, capturing all pertinent QOL information is a challenge for clinicians and researchers. Questionnaires alone cannot completely capture a patient's true feelings. Scores achieved through questionnaires are unable to capture the layered richness and complexity of individual experiences. Therefore, quantitative and qualitative measures of QOL research should be employed to capture the broad range of experiences among men with prostate cancer. Furthermore, clinicians who use QOL research must not only consider findings from quantitative and qualitative research but also must couple them with true engagement of the patient in conversation that will result in an understanding of that individual's needs, desires, and goals (Albaugh & Hacker, 2008).

Another consideration when measuring QOL is the timing of when to do so. Typically, this is determined by clinical

Figure 6-3. Quality-of-Life Questionnaires

Generic Questionnaires
- The Beck Depression Inventory (BDI)
- Functional Assessment of Cancer Therapy—General Scale (FACT-G)
- Global Adjustment to Illness Scale
- International Index of Erectile Function (IIEF) Questionnaire
- International Prostate Symptom Score (IPSS) Questionnaire
- McCorkle and Young Symptom Distress Scale
- McMaster Health Index Questionnaire
- Medical Outcome Study Short-Form General Health Survey (MOS)
- Nottingham Health Profile
- Profile of Mood States (POMS)
- Psychosocial Adjustment to Medical Illness (PAIS)
- Quality of Life Index by Padilla et al. (QLI)
- Quality of Life Index by Spitzer et al. (QL-Index)
- Rectal Function Assessment Study (R-FAS) Tool
- Schedule for the Evaluation of Individual Quality of Life-Direct Weight (SEIQOL-DW)
- Sickness Impact Profile (SIP)
- Ware Health Perceptions Questionnaire
- Bem Sex-Role Inventory—Short Form (BSRI-S)
- Importance of Sex-Role Identity (ISRI)

Cancer-Specific Questionnaires
- Cancer Rehabilitation Evaluation System (CARES)
- European Organization for Research and Treatment of Cancer (EORTC) Quality of Life Questionnaire (QLQ-C30) and QLQ-PR25 prostate cancer module
- Functional Assessment of Cancer Therapy Scale (FACT-P) module for prostate cancer
- Functional Living Index: Cancer (FLIC)
- Quality Adjusted Time Without Symptoms or Toxicity (QA "TWIST")
- Quality of life Index: Cancer Version, by Ferrans and Powers
- Southwest Oncology Group Quality of Life Questionnaire
- Southwest Oncology Group Prostate Treatment Specific Symptoms Measure (PTSS)
- The UCLA Prostate Cancer Index
- Time Without Symptoms or Toxicity (TWIST)

Note. From "Quality of Life and Prostate Cancer," by C.R. King in J. Held-Warmkessel (Ed.), *Contemporary Issues in Prostate Cancer* (2nd ed., p. 323), 2006, Sudbury, MA: Jones and Bartlett. Copyright 2006 by Jones and Bartlett. Reprinted with permission. Also based on information from Wettergren et al., 2005; Willener & Hantikained, 2005.

practice or one's research question. Patients may take several months to years to fully recover from or become psychologically adjusted to physical changes experienced following interventions aimed at treating prostate cancer. Talcott et al. (2003) supported allowing a minimal time frame of 24 months after treatment when trying to compare treatment outcomes between prostatectomy and RT. If measuring psychological implications alone, interval measurements taken over several years may be more appropriate (Albaugh & Hacker, 2008). For specific recent nursing studies that examine QOL issues in prostate cancer survivors, refer to Chapter 7 of this text.

Oncology nurses' perceived clinical utility of QOL measurement in general is another important factor. King, Hinds, Dow, Schum, and Lee (2002) found that oncology nurses reported formal QOL assessment tools to be of minimal importance. Instead, the nurses felt that the nurse-patient relationship is a more important means for assessing QOL. Despite limitations in assessing QOL, nurses attempt, whether formally or otherwise, to gauge patient perceptions and concerns as they relate to one's overall well-being. Information gained through QOL assessment should be used toward appropriate intervention and support of patients and caregivers.

Palliative Care and Hospice

In most cases, prostate cancer is now considered a chronic disease. Patients with advanced chronic disease may develop problems such as cachexia, spinal cord compression, bone pain, and bone fractures from metastatic deposits. Management of these symptoms often requires intervention from palliative care or hospice services. Palliative care no longer solely focuses on providing physical comfort to dying patients. The scope of palliative care has expanded to include managing the physical, social, psychological, and spiritual aspects of coping with the disease across the continuum of cancer care. Patients with advanced or recurrent prostate cancer need not be faced with a decision between palliation of symptoms or no treatment at all while enrolled in an end-of-life program. The goal of palliative care is to control the disease for as long as possible and effectively manage symptoms. Hospice is an integral part of palliative care. Patients with prostate cancer who have six months or less to live can be enrolled in hospice to maximize the patient's QOL. Additionally, hospice provides emotional, spiritual, and educational support for patients and families. One important component of hospice is anticipatory grieving and bereavement follow-up that caregivers and family members receive. Hospice care can be given in the patient's home, in a freestanding hospice facility, or in an inpatient/nursing home setting. Patients with advanced prostate cancer and their families should be informed of the benefits of hospice and palliative care and what each one entails, along with reinforcement that living with advanced prostate cancer does not involve an either/or choice (Crowley, 2005).

The Edmonton Symptom Assessment System (ESAS) (Capital Health, 2001) is a tool designed to assist in the assessment of nine symptoms common in patients with cancer: pain, tiredness, nausea, depression, anxiety, drowsiness, decreased or increased appetite, decreased well-being, and shortness of breath. These symptoms may be present as patients with advanced disease approach death. Therefore, this tool often is used in the palliative care and hospice setting. The patient rates the severity of symptoms at the time of the assessment using a 0–10 scale. Zero is indicative of an absence of symptoms, and a score of 10 indicates the worst possible severity of a symptom. As a result of limited clinical and research utility of the ESAS specific to definitions and terminology, subsequent revisions of the tool have been suggested (Fainsinger et al., 2005; Nekolaichuk, Fainsinger, & Lawlor, 2005). The ESAS or a revision thereof is helpful in tracking symptom severity over time and should be used as a component of a holistic clinical assessment. The ESAS or a similar type of assessment tool should be used during each palliative visit or telephone call.

Pain occurs in approximately 80%–90% of patients during the terminal phases of the disease (Chiu, Hu, & Chen, 2000; Potter, Hami, Bryan, & Quigley, 2003). One common issue for patients with advanced disease is pain related to bone metastasis. Prostate cancer cells that become hormone-independent tend to be highly invasive and are associated with an increased incidence of skeletal metastases as the disease progresses. Prostate cancer is unique in that bone often is the only clinically detectable site of metastasis, and the resulting tumors tend to be osteoblastic, which is bone-forming, rather than osteolytic, which is bone-lysing. The involvement of the skeleton by metastatic prostate cells occurs in a predictable manner, with lesions tending to appear first in the axial skeleton and subsequently in the appendicular skeleton (Logothetis & Lin, 2005). For some patients with metastatic disease to a limited number of bony sites, bisphosphonate therapy may be helpful. Bisphosphonates work by binding to bone and inhibiting osteoclastic activity and proliferation. These agents act to disrupt the cycle of bone breakdown that occurs in metastatic disease. Most men with advanced disease will have received ADT at some point as part of their overall disease management, which further increases their susceptibility to fractures (NCCN, 2008c). One study in patients with advanced disease who received bisphosphonate therapy reported a 25% reduction in the number of patients who incurred skeletal related events. The time period to the first skeletal-related event was 100 days later than in patients receiving placebo (Saad et al., 2002).

Pain from bone metastasis can be very challenging. Pain can have different meanings for patients with advanced cancer. Men in one study perceived the presence of pain as a threat of dying in agony (Lindqvist, Widmark, & Rasmussen, 2006). Patients should be instructed to report new onset of pain and the point at which currently existing pain management strategies are no longer effective. It is important to manage pain. Chronic pain frequently is managed with long-acting opioid analgesics with shorter-acting agents used for breakthrough pain (Crowley, 2005). In some cases, radiopharmaceuticals may be used to relieve ongoing chronic bony pain from metastatic prostate cancer. Agents such as strontium and samarium are used for this indication and act by chemically inhibiting the build-up of metastatic deposits on or inside the bone. For more detailed information about the use of radiopharmaceuticals for skeletal metastasis, refer to Chapters 4 and 5.

Nonpharmacologic pain relief methods can be extremely beneficial adjuncts to pharmacologic interventions for chronic pain management. Nonpharmacologic methods include physical modalities and cognitive modalities. Physical modalities include massage; physical therapy; heat or ice; acupuncture; acupressure; bed, bath, or walking supports; and positioning. Cognitive modalities include imagery, hypnosis, distraction training, relaxation training, cognitive behavioral training, and spiritual care (NCCN, 2008a).

Another method of pain control for advanced metastatic prostate cancer is RT. However, the pain relief rates reported from clinical anecdotes and randomized trials vary widely. Unfortunately, an ideal treatment administration schedule has yet to be established. Literature supports the use of single-fraction (treatment) RT in controlling bone pain related to metastasis, and yet additional literature supports multifractionation RT, so no consensus has been reached at this time (Sze, Shelley, Held, & Mason, 2004). Single-fraction dose is generally 8 gray (Gy) in one treatment, whereas a multifractionation schedule consists of a total dose of 20–30 Gy given over 4–10 fractions (Ratanatharathorn, Powers, & Temple, 2004). These treatments are given directly to the bony site of pain. Sometimes an osteolytic or osteoblastic lesion can be seen on a plain x-ray film, or correlation with a radionuclide bone scan may be necessary. Once the site to be treated is isolated, a small surrounding margin of a few centimeters is included in the treatment field. Often, RT is used in conjunction with opioid analgesics to achieve maximum pain control. On occasion, osteolytic lesions can deteriorate the structural integrity of a weight-bearing bone to the point where surgical placement of rods, pins, or plates may be indicated to stabilize the area of concern.

Wellness Care

In addition to ongoing follow-up visits with oncology team members, such as the urologist, surgical oncologist, radiation oncologist, medical oncologist, or advanced practice nurse or oncology nurse, men should partner with their primary care physician to continue (or begin) healthy lifestyle maintenance. This includes dietary modifications, exercise, and age-appropriate cancer screenings. The primary care physician resumes the coordination of care in the survivorship period. Nurses can help to educate patients about the importance of healthy lifestyle behaviors and maintaining a regular cancer screening schedule, including PSA testing and digital rectal examinations, as well as other health-related tests such as blood glucose, blood pressure, cholesterol, colorectal screening, testicular exam, eye exam, and dental exam. Education about modifiable risk factors for cancer, such as tobacco and alcohol use, is essential (Agency for Healthcare Research and Quality, 2007). Information about these and other modifiable risk factors can be obtained from the American Cancer Society (www.cancer.org).

Conclusion

Because prostate cancer is the most frequently diagnosed cancer in men, the number of men living with this disease is increasing. Oncology nurses are in an ideal position to assess for, educate about, and proactively manage late treatment effects. In addition, a proactive approach will lessen the burden of symptoms and improve QOL at any stage of the disease. Long-term effects of treatment are not limited to those of a physical nature. They also include psychosocial, spiritual, and economic concerns. Regular long-term follow-up and early intervention are key. Patients and families who know what to expect are better prepared to quickly report and manage late effects should they occur.

References

Abuaisha, B.B., Costanzi, J.B., & Boulton, A.J. (1998). Acupuncture for the treatment of chronic painful peripheral diabetic neuropathy: A long-term study. *Diabetes Research and Clinical Practice, 39*(2), 115–121.

Agency for Healthcare Research and Quality. (2007, February). *Men: Stay healthy at any age.* Retrieved September 30, 2007, from http://www.ahrq.gov/ppip/healthymen.htm

Ahmed, S., & Davies, J. (2005). Managing the complications of prostate cryosurgery. *BJU International, 95*(4), 480–481.

Albaugh, J., & Hacker, E.D. (2008). Measurement of quality of life in men with prostate cancer. *Clinical Journal of Oncology Nursing, 12*(1), 81–86.

American Cancer Society. (2008). *Cancer facts and figures, 2008.* Retrieved March 15, 2008, from http://www.cancer.org/downloads/STT/2008CAFFfinalsecured.pdf

Armstrong, T., Almadrones, T., & Gilbert, M.R. (2005). Chemotherapy-induced peripheral neuropathy. *Oncology Nursing Forum, 32*(2), 305–311.

Ashman, J.B., Zelefsky, M.J., Hunt, M.S., Leibel, S.A., & Fuks, Z. (2005). Whole pelvic radiotherapy for prostate cancer using 3D conformal and intensity-modulated radiotherapy. *International Journal of Radiation Oncology, Biology, Physics, 63*(3), 765–771.

Barry, M.J., Fowler, F.J., O'Leary, M.P., Bruskewitz, R.C., Holtgrewe, H.L., Mebust, W.K., et al. (1992). The American Urological Association symptom index for benign prostatic hyperplasia: The measurement committee of the American Urological Association. *Journal of Urology, 148*(5), 1549–1557.

Basaria, S., Lieb, J., Tang, A.M., DeWeese, T., Carducci, M., Eisenberger, M., et al. (2002). Long-term effects of androgen deprivation therapy in prostate cancer patients. *Clinical Endocrinology, 56*(6), 779–786.

Bedford Laboratories. (2004). *Cisplatin injection* [Package insert]. Bedford, OH: Author. Retrieved February 8, 2008, from http://www.bedfordlabs.com/products/inserts/CIS-AQ-P01.pdf

Bellizzi, K.M., Latini, D.M., Cowan, J.E., DuChane, J., & Carroll, P.R. (2006). *Fear of recurrence, symptom burden and quality of life in men with prostate cancer: A prospective analysis from CaPSURE.* Poster session presented at the 2006 Prostate Cancer Symposium of the American Society of Clinical Oncology, Atlanta, GA. Retrieved March 14, 2008, from http://urology.ucsf.edu/capsure/abs/abs.aspx

Blank, T.O., & Bellizzi, K.M. (2006). After prostate cancer: Predictors of well being among long-term cancer survivors. *Cancer, 106*(10), 2128–2134.

Brown, M.W., Brooks, J.P., Albert, P.S., & Poggi, M.M. (2007). An analysis of erectile function after intensity modulated radiation therapy for localized prostate carcinoma. *Prostate Cancer and Prostatic Diseases, 10*(2), 189–193.

Brunelli, B., & Gorson, K.C. (2004). The use of complementary and alternative medicines by patients with peripheral neuropathy. *Journal of Neurological Sciences, 218*(1–2), 59–66.

Bruner, D.W., Haas, M.L., & Gosselin-Acomb, T.K. (Eds.). (2005). *Manual for radiation oncology nursing practice and education* (3rd ed.). Pittsburgh, PA: Oncology Nursing Society.

Capital Health. (2001). *Guidelines for using the Edmonton Symptom Assessment System (ESAS).* Retrieved September 27, 2007, from http://www.palliative.org/PC/ClinicalInfo/AssessmentTools/esas.pdf

Carpenter, J.S. (2001). The hot flash related daily interference scale: A tool for assessing the impact of hot flashes on quality of life following breast cancer. *Journal of Pain and Symptom Management, 22*(6), 979–989.

Cella, D.F., Tulsky, D.S., Gray, G., Sarafian, B., Linn, E., Bonomi, A., et al. (1993). The Functional Assessment of Cancer Therapy Scale: Development and validation of the general measure. *Journal of Clinical Oncology, 11*(3), 570–579.

Chiu, T.Y., Hu, W.Y., & Chen, C.Y. (2000). Prevalence and severity of symptoms in terminal cancer patients: A study in Taiwan. *Supportive Care in Oncology, 8*(4), 311–313.

Clark, J.A., & Talcott, J.A. (2006). Confidence and uncertainty long after initial treatment for early prostate cancer: Survivors' views of cancer control and the treatment decisions they made. *Journal of Clinical Oncology, 24*(27), 4457–4463.

Crowley, M.J. (2005). Supportive care: Dying and death. In J.K. Itano & K.N. Taoka (Eds.), *Core curriculum for oncology nursing* (4th ed., pp. 102–107). St. Louis, MO: Elsevier Saunders.

Daubenmier, J.J., Weidner, G., Marlin, R., Crutchfield, L., Dunn-Emke, S., Chi, C., et al. (2005). Lifestyle and health-related quality of life of men with prostate cancer managed with active surveillance. *Adult Urology, 67*(1), 125–130.

DeMeerleer, G.O., Fonteyne, V.H., Vakaet, L., Villeirs, G.M., Denoyette, L., Varbaeys, A., et al. (2007). Intensity-modulated radiation therapy for prostate cancer: Late morbidity and results on biochemical control. *Radiotherapy and Oncology, 82*(2), 160–166.

Fainsinger, R.L., Nekolaichuk, C.L., Lawlor, P.G., Neumann, C.M., Hanson, J., & Vigano, A. (2005). A multicenter study of the revised Edmonton Staging System for classifying cancer pain in advanced cancer patients. *Journal of Symptom Management, 29*(3), 224–237.

Ferrell, B.R., Dow, K.H., & Grant, M. (1995). Measurement of the quality of life in cancer survivors. *Quality of Life Research, 4*(6), 523–531.

Fortner, B., Okon, T., Ashley, J., Kepler, G., Chavez, J., Tauer, K., et al. (2003). The Zero Acceptance of Pain (ZAP) Quality Improvement Project: Evaluation of pain severity pain interference, global quality of life, and pain-related costs. *Journal of Pain and Symptom Management, 25*(4), 334–343.

Fortenbaugh, C.C., & Rummel, M.A. (2007). *Case studies in oncology nursing: Text and review.* Sudbury, MA: Jones and Bartlett.

Ganzer, H., & Selle, C. (2006). Improving reimbursement for oncology nutrition services. *Oncology Issues, 9,* 34–37.

Geinitz, H., Zimmerman, F., Thamm, R., Erber, C., Muller, T., Keller, M., et al. (2006). Late rectal symptoms and quality of life after conformal radiation therapy for prostate cancer. *Radiotherapy and Oncology, 79*(3), 341–347.

Guise, T.A., Oefelein, M.G., Eastham, J.A., Cookson, M.S., Higano, C.S., & Smith, M.R. (2007). Estrogenic side effects of androgen deprivation therapy. *Reviews in Urology, 9*(4), 163–180.

Haylock, P.J., Mitchell, S.A., Cox, T., Temple, S.V., & Curtiss, C.P. (2007). The cancer survivor's prescription for living: Nurses must take the lead in planning care for survivors. *American Journal of Nursing, 107*(4), 58–70.

Hewitt, M.E., Greenfield, S., & Stovall, E. (Eds.). (2005). *From cancer patient to cancer survivor: Lost in transition* (pp. 187–321). Washington, DC: National Academies Press.

Hogle, W.P. (2007). Male genitourinary cancers. In M.L. Haas, W.P. Hogle, G.J. Moore-Higgs, & T.K. Gosselin-Acomb (Eds.), *Radiation therapy: A guide to patient care* (pp. 234–248). St. Louis, MO: Mosby.

Hunter, K.F., Moore, K.N., & Glazener, C.M. (2007). Conservative management for postprostatectomy urinary incontinence. *Cochrane Database of Systematic Reviews* 2007, Issue 1. Art. No.: CD001843. DOI: 10.1002/14651858.CD001843.pub3.

Hyacinth, J.J., Thibault, G.P., & Ruttle-King, J. (2006). Perceived stress and quality of life among prostate cancer survivors. *Military Journal, 171*(5), 425–429.

Incrocci, L., Slob, A.K., & Levendag, P.C. (2002). Sexual (dys)function after radiotherapy for prostate cancer: A review. *International Journal of Radiation Oncology, Biology, Physics, 52*(3), 681–693.

Israeli, R.S., Ryan, C.W., & Jung, L.L. (2008). Managing bone loss in men with locally advanced prostate cancer receiving androgen deprivation therapy. *Journal of Urology, 179*(2), 414–423.

Jemal, A., Siegel, R., Ward, E., Hao, Y., Xu, J., Murray, T., et al. (2008). Cancer statistics, 2008. *CA: A Cancer Journal for Clinicians, 58*(2), 71–96.

Johnson, G.D., Moore, K., & Fortner, B. (2007). Baseline evaluation of the AIM Higher initiative: Establishing the mark from which to measure. *Oncology Nursing Forum, 34*(3), 729–734.

Kattan, M. (2006). Measuring hot flashes in men treated with hormone ablation therapy: An unmet need. *Urologic Nursing, 26*(1), 13–18.

King, C.R. (2006). Quality of life and prostate cancer. In J. Held-Warmkessel (Ed.), *Contemporary issues in prostate cancer* (2nd ed., pp. 318–352). Sudbury, MA: Jones and Bartlett.

King, C.R., Hinds, P.S., Dow, K.H., Schum, B.A., & Lee, C.K. (2002). The nurse's relationship-based perceptions of patient quality of life [Online exclusive]. *Oncology Nursing Forum, 29*(10), E118–E126. Retrieved August 20, 2007, from http://ons.metapress.com/content/d242m4020t767760/fulltext.pdf

Lindqvist, O., Widmark, A., & Rasmussen, B. (2006). Reclaiming wellness-living with bodily problems, as narrated by men with advanced prostate cancer. *Cancer Nursing, 29*(4), 327–337.

Logothetis, C.J., & Lin, S. (2005). Osteoblasts in prostate cancer metastasis to bone. *Nature Reviews: Cancer, 5*(1), 21–28.

Loprinzi, C.L, Khoyratty, B.S., Dueck, A., Barton, D.L., Jafar, S., Rowland, K.M., et al. (2007). Gabapentin for hot flashes in men: NCCTG trial N00CB. *Journal of Clinical Oncology, 25*(Suppl. 18), Abstract 9005.

Moore, S. (2004). Menopausal symptoms. In C.H. Yarbro, M.H. Frogge, & M. Goodman (Eds.), *Cancer symptom management* (3rd ed., pp. 571–590). Sudbury, MA: Jones and Bartlett.

Nandipati, K.C., Raina, R., Agarwal, A., & Zippe, C.D. (2007). Nerve-sparing surgery significantly affects long-term continence after radical prostatectomy. *Urology, 70*(6), 1127–1130.

National Cancer Institute. (2006). *Common terminology criteria for adverse events* (Version 3.0). Retrieved March 14, 2008, from http://ctep.cancer.gov/forms/CTCAEv3.pdf

National Cancer Institute. (2007). *Clinical trials: Prostate cancer.* Retrieved August 20, 2007, from http://www.cancer.gov/search/ResultsClinicalTrialsAdvanced.aspx?protocolsearchid=4372165

National Comprehensive Cancer Network. (2007). *NCCN Clinical Practice Guidelines in Oncology™. Distress management* [v.1.2008]. Retrieved July 21, 2008, from http://www.nccn.org/professionals/physician_gls/PDF/distress.pdf

National Comprehensive Cancer Network. (2008a). *NCCN Clinical Practice Guidelines in Oncology™. Adult cancer pain* [v.1.2008]. Retrieved July 21, 2008, from http://www.nccn.org/professionals/physician_gls/PDF/pain.pdf

National Comprehensive Cancer Network. (2008b). *NCCN Clinical Practice Guidelines in Oncology™. Cancer-related fatigue* [v.1.2008]. Retrieved July 21, 2008, from http://www.nccn.org/professionals/physician_gls/PDF/fatigue.pdf

National Comprehensive Cancer Network. (2008c). *NCCN Clinical Practice Guidelines in Oncology™. Prostate cancer* [v.2.2007]. Retrieved July 21, 2008, from http://www.nccn.org/professionals/physician_gls/PDF/prostate.pdf

Nekolaichuk, C.L., Fainsinger, R.L., & Lawlor, P.G. (2005). A validation study of a pain classification system for advanced cancer patients using content experts: The Edmonton Classification System for Cancer Pain. *Palliative Medicine, 19*(6), 466–476.

Nitti, V.W., Kim, Y., & Combs, A.J. (1994). Correlation of the AUA symptom index with urodynamics in patients with suspected benign prostatic hyperplasia. *Neurourology and Urodynamics, 13*(5), 521–529.

Otto, S.E. (2004). *Oncology nursing clinical reference.* St. Louis, MO: Mosby.

Ottery, F.D. (2000). Patient-Generated Subjective Global Assessment. In P.D. McCallum & C.G. Polisena (Eds.), *The clinical guide to oncology nutrition* (pp. 11–23). Chicago: American Dietetic Association.

O'Connel, B., Baker, L., & Munro, I. (2007). The nature and impact of incontinence in men who have undergone prostate surgery and implications for nursing practice. *Contemporary Nurse, 24*(1), 65–78.

O'Rourke, M.E. (2005). Nursing care. In J.K. Itano & K.N. Taoka (Eds.), *Core curriculum for oncology nursing* (4th ed., pp. 610–611). St. Louis, MO: Elsevier Saunders.

Owen, J.E., Goldstein, M.S., Lee, J.H., Breen, N., & Rowland, J.H. (2007). Use of health-related and cancer-specific support groups among adult cancer survivors. *Cancer, 109*(12), 2580–2589.

Petrylak, D., Tangen, C., Hussain, M., Lara, P., Jones, J., Taplin, M., et al. (2004). Docetaxel and estramustine compared with mitoxantrone and prednisone for advanced refractory prostate cancer. *New England Journal of Medicine, 351*(15), 1513–1520.

Polovich, M., White, J.M., & Kelleher, L.M. (Eds.). (2005). *Chemotherapy and biotherapy guidelines and recommendations for practice* (2nd ed.). Pittsburgh, PA: Oncology Nursing Society.

Potter, J., Hami, F., Bryan, T., & Quigley, C. (2003). Symptoms in 400 patients referred to palliative care services: Prevalence and patterns. *Palliative Medicine, 17*(4), 310–314.

Ratanatharathorn, V., Powers, W.E., & Temple, H.T. (2004). Palliation of bone metastases. In C.A. Perez, L.W. Brady, E.C. Halperin, & R.K. Schmidt-Ullrich (Eds.), *Principles and practice of radiation oncology* (4th ed., pp. 2385–2404). Philadelphia: Lippincott Williams & Wilkins.

Reeve, B.B., Potosky, A.L., & Willis, G.B. (2006). Should function and bother be measured and reported separately for prostate cancer quality-of-life domains? *Adult Urology, 79*(3), 341–347.

Rutledge, D.N., & McGuire, C. (2004). Evidence-based symptom management. In C.H. Yarbro, M.H. Frogge, & M. Goodman (Eds.), *Cancer symptom management* (3rd ed., pp. 3–14). Sudbury, MA: Jones and Bartlett.

Saad, F., Gleason, D.M., Murray, R., Tchekmedyian, S., Venner, P., Lacombe, L., et al. (2002). A randomized, placebo-controlled trial of zoledronic acid in patients with hormone-refractory metastatic prostate carcinoma. *Journal of the National Cancer Institute, 94*(19), 1458–1468.

Sanders, S., Pedro, L.W., Bantum, E.O., & Galbraith, M.E. (2006). Couples surviving prostate cancer: Long-term intimacy needs and concerns following treatment. *Clinical Journal of Oncology Nursing, 10*(4), 503–508.

Shell, J.A. (2007). Sexuality and sexual dysfunction. In M.L. Haas, W.P. Hogle, G.J. Moore-Higgs, & T.K. Gosselin-Acomb (Eds.), *Radiation therapy: A guide to patient care* (3rd ed., pp. 609–623). St. Louis, MO: Mosby.

Shu, H.G., Lee, T.T., Vigneauly, E., Xia, P., Pickett, B., Phillips, T.L., et al. (2001). Toxicity following high dose three-dimensional conformal and intensity modulated radiation therapy for clinically localized prostate cancer. *Urology, 57*(1), 102–107.

Sze, W.M., Shelley, M., Held, I., & Mason, M. (2004). Palliation of metastatic bone pain: Single fraction versus multifraction radiotherapy. *Cochrane Database of Systematic Reviews* 2002, Issue 1. Art. No.: CD004721. DOI: 10.1002/14651858.CD004721.

Talcott, J.A., Manola, J., Clark, J.A., Kaplan, I., Beard, C.J., Mitchel, S.P., et al. (2003). Time course and predictors of symptoms after primary prostate cancer therapy. *Journal of Clinical Oncology, 21*(21), 3979–3986.

Tannock, I., de Witt, R., Berry, W.R., Horti, J., Pluzanska, A., Chi, K.N., et al. (2004). Docetaxel plus prednisone or mitoxantrone plus prednisone for advanced prostate cancer. *New England Journal of Medicine, 351*(15), 1502–1512.

Taylor, L.C., Demoor, C., Smith, M.A., Dunn, A.L., Basen-Engquist, K., Nielsen, I., et al. (2006). Active for life after cancer: A randomized trial examining a lifestyle physical activity program for prostate cancer patients. *Psycho-Oncology, 15*(10), 847–862.

Tewari, A., Peabody, J., Sarle, R., Balakrisnan, G., Hemal, A., Shrivastava, A., et al. (2002). Technique of da Vinci robot-assisted anatomic radical prostatectomy. *Urology, 60*(4), 569–572.

Thompson, C.A., Shanafelt, T.D., & Loprinzi, C.L. (2003). Andropause: Symptom management for prostate cancer patients treated with hormonal ablation. *Oncologist, 8*(5), 474–487.

Ward, S.E., Goldberg, N., Miller-McCauley, V., Meuller, C., Nolan, A., Pawlik-Plank, D., et al. (1993). Patient-related barriers to management of cancer pain. *Pain, 52*(3), 319–324.

Weintraub, M.I., Wolfe, G.I., Barohn, R.A., Cole, S.P., Parry, G.J., Hayat, G., et al. (2003). Static magnetic field therapy for symptomatic diabetic neuropathy: A randomized, double-blind, placebo-controlled trial. *Archives of Physical Medicine and Rehabilitation, 84*(5), 736–746.

Wilkes, G.M., & Barton-Burke, M. (2007). *2007 oncology nursing drug handbook.* Sudbury, MA: Jones and Bartlett.

Wettergren, L., Björkholm, M., & Langius-Eklöf, A. (2005). Validation of an extended version of the SEIQoL-DW in a cohort of Hodgkin lymphoma survivors. *Quality of Life Research, 14*(10), 2329–2333.

Yellen, S.B., Cella, D.F., Webster, K., Blendowski, C., & Kaplan, E. (1997). Measuring fatigue and other anemia-related symptoms with the Functional Assessment of Cancer Therapy (FACT) measurement system. *Journal of Pain and Symptom Management, 13*(2), 63–74.

Zelefsky, M.J., Cowen, D., Fuks, Z., Shike, M., Burman, C., Jackson, A., et al. (1999). Long term tolerance of high dose three-dimensional conformal radiotherapy in patients with localized prostate carcinoma. *Cancer, 85*(11), 2460–2468.

Zelefsky, M.J., Fuks, Z., Hunt, M., Yamada, Y., Marion, C., Ling, C.C., et al. (2002). High dose intensity modulated radiation therapy for prostate cancer: Early toxicity and biochemical outcome in 772 patients. *International Journal of Radiation Oncology, Biology, Physics, 53*(5), 1111–1116.

CHAPTER 7

Nursing Research Contributions to the Care of Patients With Prostate Cancer

Tracy K. Gosselin, RN, MSN, PhD(c), AOCN®

Introduction

Care of men diagnosed with prostate cancer represents a multidimensional construct that is influenced by a variety of factors, which may include age, staging, treatment, symptom management, and social support. Nursing research is a critical component of the advancement of nursing knowledge and offers researchers and clinicians opportunities for collaboration. As other chapters in this book have highlighted prevention, staging, treatment, survivorship, and nursing care, it must be noted that advancements from nursing research have influenced many of these areas directly and indirectly.

The purpose of this chapter is to highlight the contributions of nursing research as well as to identify gaps and future directions. This chapter is not meant to provide the reader with a comprehensive overview of all studies reported in the literature but rather an understanding of the diversity of nursing research related to prostate cancer. This chapter will include nursing research studies from the eight-year period of 2000–2007 that may be qualitative or quantitative, from the United States and other countries (see Table 7-1). A variety of search engines were used to identify scholarly work, and search terms included *prostate cancer, nurs-ing,* and *research* as well as *prostate cancer and nursing research*. A variety of nursing and non-nursing journals are represented. The Oncology Nursing Society's (ONS's) 2005–2009 research agenda identified the following six content areas (ONS, 2005).

- Cancer symptoms and side effects
- Individual- and family-focused psychosocial and behavioral research
- Health promotion focusing on primary and secondary prevention
- Late effects of cancer treatment and long-term survivorship issues for patients and families
- Research that looks at nursing-sensitive patient outcomes
- Translational research to develop, test, and evaluate strategies designed to determine which system- and clinician-related factors affect the clinical application of already-created evidence-based guidelines

These content areas will be used to structure this chapter. The areas of nursing-sensitive patient outcomes and translational research will not be highlighted, as identified articles did not fall into these topic areas.

Health Promotion: Primary and Secondary Prevention

Prevention and screening for prostate cancer has gained significant attention over the past 10 years. Although no nursing prevention studies were found related to prevention, the significant impact that nurses had in the conduct and facilitation of the Prostate Cancer Prevention Trial (PCPT) (www.cancer.gov/pcpt) and the Selenium and Vitamin E Cancer Prevention Trial (SELECT) (www.crab.org/select) must be considered. Combined, the studies accrued more than 50,000 men. Results from the PCPT are available, whereas final results from the SELECT study will not be available for several years.

Screening for prostate cancer, which includes digital rectal examination (DRE) and prostate-specific antigen (PSA)

Table 7-1. Information on Studies Included	
Type of Study/Country	Number of Studies
Qualitative	9
Quantitative	13
Country	
Australia	1
Canada	5
Sweden	2
Switzerland	1
United Kingdom	2
United States	11

testing which remains a controversial topic in the literature (Ilic, O'Connor, Green, & Wilt, 2006; Oliffe, 2006). Primary prevention focuses on what one does to prevent disease from happening, whereas secondary prevention focuses on early detection. Nursing articles in this area focused on secondary prevention. Meade, Calvo, Rivera, and Baer (2003) used focus groups to understand Hispanic farm workers and African American males' everyday concerns in the development of cancer screening education materials. The researchers developed a focus group interview guide and recruited a total of 71 participants to four focus groups. Men were noted to have a general lack of knowledge about prostate cancer but identified that spokespeople should include cancer survivors, doctors as experts, and community leaders. Themes that developed during the interviews led to the development of two culturally appropriate prostate cancer educational toolboxes.

Kleier (2006) conducted another study addressing the need for a culturally diverse questionnaire. In a descriptive study, this researcher reviewed the process that took place to translate the Prostate Health Questionnaire for Jamaican and Haitian men into three different dialects. The translation process, the teams that were brought together, validation, and testing for internal consistency were all reviewed. A total of 156 men (69 Jamaican, 87 Haitian) completed the translated instrument, with some completing it an additional time for test-retest. The translated instrument was found to be comprehensive, to have internal consistency, and to have high stability over time. Both groups were found to be equally insured for health care, yet only 50.6% of Haitian men had ever been screened for prostate cancer, compared to 72.5% of Jamaican men. Results of this study support the need for culturally appropriate instruments and also the need for education of men who should be screened for prostate cancer.

A qualitative study by Oliffe (2006) used semistructured interviews and participant observation to describe the experience of prostate cancer screening and subsequent cancer diagnosis. Thirty-five participants were recruited from prostate cancer support groups or from advertisements in newspapers. Four categories were identified, each with thematic findings. The first category was *Prescreen: Screening Reason*, which had two themes—physical symptoms and testimonials. Sixty percent of participants experienced lower urinary tract symptoms and related these symptoms to lifestyle or advanced age, with some participants monitoring them for a long amount of time before consulting a general practitioner (GP). Spousal influence directly affected 17.14% of the participants in seeing a GP, whereas only 14.28% had awareness of prostate cancer from a family member or friend. The next category was *Screening: Preferences and Patterns*, which had three themes. Researchers found that participants preferred PSA testing over DRE. One participant stated, "I had to gear myself up [for the DRE]." When the GP recommended screening, 88% recalled having little or no understanding of PSA screening. The third category focused on *Abnormal Results: The Whiff of Bedlam*.

Participants revealed the stress they experienced and the steps that were put into motion once it was determined they had an elevated PSA level. The final category was *Prostate Cancer Diagnosis: Shock and Treatment*. Of the participants, 16.66% sought a second opinion, and 91.66% were treated by the specialist to whom they were referred. The role of androgen deprivation therapy in patients with advanced cancer was noted to "starve the tumor" and "allow me to finish projects." This study shed light on the fact that many men did not know that three different tests are needed to confirm a diagnosis of prostate cancer and also informed nurses about what men are thinking as they are going through this process.

A Solomon Four research design study was conducted to evaluate an enhanced decision aid versus a usual care decision aid in men deciding on prostate cancer screening (Weinrich, Seger, et al., 2007). This study design controls for pretest measures, as it is believed that pretest questions could influence intervention and post-test responses. A total of 198 men were randomized to one of four groups, with 78% of the sample being African American and 52% being low income. The primary author of this article developed the enhanced decision aid, which included a variety of concepts pertinent to prostate screening and was 12 pages long. The usual care aid was two pages long and was developed by the American Cancer Society. Taking the pretest was found to increase post-test scores regardless of which decision aid was used, especially in men who had undergone previous DRE (p = .02). Additionally, higher educational level and income were significant predictors of knowledge scores. At the end of the study, all men decided to be screened, and 16% had abnormal screening results.

The impact of genetic discoveries over the past few decades has led researchers and clinicians down a new road of health promotion, education, counseling, and treatment, especially in high-risk populations. Weinrich, Vijayakumar, et al. (2007) studied hereditary prostate cancer knowledge in 79 African American men who had four or more family members with a diagnosis of prostate cancer. Researchers conducted telephone interviews and assessed knowledge with the nine-item Knowledge of Hereditary Prostate Cancer Scale. Results showed that questions related to genetic susceptibility were most likely to be answered incorrectly or not at all, whereas those related to inheritance were answered correctly by more than half. Furthermore, 82% of respondents were able to correctly answer the question "Men are more likely to get prostate cancer if they have three or more family members with prostate cancer." Interestingly, men without prostate cancer had a higher percentage of correct responses to this question. Age was found to be a predictor of knowledge (p = .002), with older men being more knowledgeable. Additionally, a high percentage of respondents did not answer the question related to risk probability and having had a positive test. In summary, the authors concluded that knowledge and education related to hereditary prostate cancer are essential for patients and family members, and healthcare providers need to stay abreast of changes in this rapidly evolving field.

Diagnosis

As identified earlier by Oliffe (2006), three tests are needed to confirm a diagnosis of prostate cancer. The last of those tests performed is a transrectal ultrasound prostate biopsy (TRUS-Bx). In an ethnographic study of 30 men who underwent TRUS-Bx, Oliffe (2004) identified two categories. The first category of *Leading Up to TRUS-Bx* identified one pattern related to anxious uncertainty. Oliffe noted that the amount of time varied from three days to six months for the procedure after the confirmation of an abnormality by PSA testing or DRE. He also noted that few men confided in their spouse or healthcare professionals about what they were feeling. The second category, *TRUS-Bx*, had three patterns. The first was related to *Anal Penetration*, and men reported mild discomfort related to insertion. *Needling Pain*, the second pattern, noted that the diverse pain and anxiety made it hard to predict a uniform patient experience. Ninety percent of men described increasing levels of anxiety and pain as the procedure continued. The final pattern was *Painless Expectations*, and men reported more discomfort than what they were led to expect. Sixty-six percent of the participants recalled being assured that they would be able to tolerate the procedure without analgesia or anesthetic, and although 90% reported pain or discomfort during the procedure, only one man reported this to the clinician.

Treatment

Treatment for prostate cancer has evolved significantly over the past 20 years. The role of multidisciplinary clinics, the advent of new radiation approaches and technology, and greater advocacy in general have led to significant improvements in overall survival. Treatment approaches entail a variety of techniques that cover the disease trajectory. A variety of surgical approaches exist, with robot-assisted devices allowing for further refinement. Radiation therapy (RT) has evolved from a four-field box to three-dimensional conformal treatment that is being further advanced with the use of intensity-modulated radiation therapy that may incorporate the use of ultrasound, personal dosimeters, and image-guided techniques. Brachytherapy approaches continue to evolve, with high-dose-rate treatments being incorporated into external beam RT. Hormonal therapy is used across the continuum to shrink the prostate initially and also in the advanced disease setting to control disease. Finally, the role of radioactive isotopes and palliative RT cannot be understated, as they are used for symptom control in patients with advanced disease.

Many men also may decide to forgo the previously described treatment options for localized prostate cancer and instead choose active surveillance (i.e., watchful waiting). In a hermeneutic phenomenologic study, Hedestig, Sandman, and Widmark (2003) explored what it meant to be a man living with untreated prostate cancer. In their analysis, four themes emerged. The first is *To Be Alone With the Disease Experience*. This theme encompassed protecting and not worrying loved ones, the perception that people prefer to stay away from those with cancer, and that these men did not want to be pitied by others. The second theme, *To Be Uncertain, Afraid, and Worried*, discovered the use of metaphors, the issues of uncertainty, and different ways of coping to manage the fear, uncertainty, and worry that accompanied watchful waiting. The next theme, *A Masculine Experience*, identified changes in manhood related to potency and ejaculation as well as difficulty in discussing sexual issues. The final theme, *The Physician—A Companion*, found that when asked about healthcare providers, the only providers mentioned were physicians. Additionally, men noted feeling safe, secure, and confidant in this relationship that was almost a friendship. This study identified many important themes for future research as well as components of care that need to be addressed.

Once a man is diagnosed is with prostate cancer, the amount of information related to the different treatments and respective side effects often can be overwhelming. In some cases, the man may not be provided with enough information to make an informed decision. In a study of 294 men, Davison, Goldenberg, Wiens, and Gleave (2007) compared a generic support program (the men watched a video on different treatments) versus an individualized decisional support program (the men used a computer program to identify information preferences) at an education center. Both groups received a standard packet of written materials and completed pretests and post-tests once a decision was made regarding treatment. Patients who received the individualized information were significantly more satisfied (p = .002) with the type, amount, and delivery method of information and their level of involvement in making a decision with the physician once a decision was made. These patients also found that the information helped them to "weigh the pros and cons of each treatment option" and "helped to prepare me to communicate my opinions" (p = .002 and p = .05, respectively) (p. E12). Overall, the individualized intervention did not result in higher levels of decisional control.

A phenomenologic study explored the lived experience of hormone ablation in 20 men (Ng, Kristjanson, & Medigovich, 2006). Data analysis identified an illness trajectory consisting of five phases, as well as two additional themes related to *Coping Strategies* and *Quality of Healthcare Relationships*. In the first phase, *Discovering the Disease*, researchers noted that participants discovered their cancer through their own preparedness, by chance, or in response to symptoms. Emotional responses included fear, panic, and shock, with one participant stating, "You first don't really understand what it is all about" (p. 208). The *Decision-Making Dilemmas* phase described how physician's preference, cost of treatment, success rate, and other patients' stories influenced decision making. The third phase, *Experiencing the Effects of Treatment*, identified three key areas: loss of sexual power, psychological changes, and physical changes. In *Living With Outcomes*, participants expressed thoughts related to acceptance, anger, and regret, with fear of death being mentioned frequently. The final phase, *Reaching Toward Health*, noted that men adopted lifestyle changes that included making dietary changes, exercising, reading, meditating, and having a positive outlook. Men also became aware of quality-of-life (QOL) choices; as one man stated, "You take a different slant in life. It makes you appreciate things more" (p. 209). The final two themes identified the use of information, family and friends, and the use of support groups as coping strategies, and supportive healthcare professionals and quality of communication were linked to quality of healthcare relationships.

In another study, researchers studied the impact of an educational intervention on men receiving hormonal manipulation therapy (Templeton & Coates, 2004). The purpose was to evaluate an evidence-based education booklet and had a pretest/post-test design. A total of 55 men completed both measures at both time points. Instruments included an investigator-developed instrument, the Functional Assessment of Cancer Therapy–Prostate (FACT-P), the Jalowiec Coping Scale, and the Client Satisfaction Questionnaire. Knowledge related to disease and hormonal treatment between groups on the pre- and post-tests was found to be significant ($p < .001$) in the experimental group, whereas no significant difference occurred in the control group. All QOL subscale measures in the experimental group were found to be significantly different at the pre- and post-test, whereas the control group only had one subscale (prostate cancer–specific concerns) that was found to be significant. The authors noted that no difference was found in either group related to coping at the time points. The authors concluded that education related to treatment improved satisfaction and knowledge related to treatment.

The final study in this area investigated the impact of external beam RT on men and the experience of living after treatment is completed (Hedestig, Sandman, Tomic, & Widmark, 2005). In this study, researchers interviewed 10 men who were at least seven months out of treatment. Upon completion of the analysis, four themes emerged. The first theme was related to *Bearing the Emotional Experience of the Illness Alone*. In this theme, men described the unwillingness to talk with others about their emotions and deepest thoughts related to the illness. Patients kept their fears, worry, and anxiety to themselves or helped to decrease these feelings by being in nature or by doing something physical. It is important to note that none of the men discussed the treatment decision with their wives. The second theme identified was *A Sense of Being Exposed*. This theme captured the essence of healthcare provider gender and

the ability to discuss physical and sexual issues. Men felt more comfortable being exposed and having discussions with male healthcare providers. The third theme, *Striving for a Sense of Having Control in a New Life Situation*, identified three different focuses, with the first being the mystery of RT. Men noted that they wanted their treatment arranged the same way every day and that some mystery exists as to how radiation works. Next was the struggle for control of disease progression, with the feeling that the PSA value is the most important piece of data received at an appointment, as it provided some sense of security. The final focus in this theme was related to a struggle for control over daily life. Men discussed the need for lifestyle adaptation and planning in advance because of bowel and urinary symptoms, which was noted to have a negative impact on QOL. The final theme, *Striving to Become Reconciled With a New Life Situation*, described the helpfulness of sharing stories with other men with prostate cancer and finding activities to shift the focus and forget about being a patient. Additionally, having the same physician and nurse throughout treatment provided a sense of security.

Cancer Symptoms and Side Effects

Symptoms of prostate cancer as well as side effects of treatment often affect QOL; however, symptoms related to these two areas require different education and intervention. Prostate cancer treatment may induce a variety of side effects that are not modality specific and yet may exacerbate the effect of one another. An example of this is men who undergo a prostatectomy who are then required to undergo RT, who then are placed at higher risk for sexual dysfunction. Patients with advanced disease may experience different symptoms related to metastatic disease and the side effects of those treatments.

Patients undergoing radical or robot-assisted prostatectomy require specific discharge teaching related to self-care and symptom management in the home setting. Managing symptoms in the home postoperatively often can be stressful for the patient and spouse. In a prospective study, researchers evaluated the impact of a discharge planning program in 100 men who underwent a radical prostatectomy (Davison, Moore, MacMillan, Bisaillon, & Wiens, 2004). The discharge program consisted of a patient education booklet (provided before the surgery), an education checklist, a discharge bag, and a telephone call at 48 hours and 30 days after discharge. The discharge bag contained urinary leg and collection bags, wound care supplies, incontinence products, and a community resource brochure. Results showed that 87% of patients had read the booklet and felt that more information was needed related to postsurgical complications, troubleshooting catheter-related problems, incision care, and incontinence related to catheter removal and pelvic floor exercises. Ninety-four percent of patients were very or moderately satisfied with the unit-based teaching, and respondents noted that catheter care was the most valuable topic of education. Furthermore, 83% of patients found the phone call 48 hours after discharge to be useful, as they felt that someone cared. Questions related to bowel management, the urinary catheter, incision care, and pain control were addressed during this call. A few respondents noted that a call between the 48-hour and 30-day call would have been beneficial. Patients found the continence and catheter supplies to be the most important items in the discharge bag. The authors also found that 25% of patients made visits to an emergency department for postdischarge problems. Overall, the authors concluded that this program had a positive impact, yet some changes would need to be considered before being incorporated into routine practice.

Side effects of hormonal therapy in patients with prostate cancer produce some similar and yet unique side effects compared to other treatment modalities. Templeton and Coates (2001) reported on their adaptation of an instrument to measure informational needs of men receiving hormonal manipulation therapy. The authors reviewed their adaptation of the Toronto Informational Needs Questionnaire that was developed for use in patients with breast cancer. The final scale had 29 questions with five categories: disease (3), physical (3), treatment (10), psychosocial (7), and integrative tests (6). The authors identified the need for evidence-based practice and how this instrument can help with the development of needed materials. Although this paper did not report final study results from the 90 men sampled, the authors did note that based on preliminary analysis, men demonstrated knowledge deficits related to disease and treatment.

Individual- and Family-Focused Psychosocial and Behavioral Research

The Institute of Medicine (2007) report *Cancer Care for the Whole Patient: Meeting Psychosocial Health Needs* identified six areas of psychosocial problems as well as services that can help to meet these identified patient care needs. The impact of a prostate cancer diagnosis extends far beyond the patient to the spouse, caregiver, and family. Studies in this section look at the impact of a prostate cancer diagnosis on the patient as well as on the spouse.

Mishel et al. (2003) looked to identify how individual characteristics of men with localized disease moderated the effects of a psychoeducational uncertainty management intervention. Mishel et al. defined uncertainty as "a fluctuating experience that never totally resolves in cancer; therefore, the purpose of intervention is not to eliminate uncertainty, but to assist patients in managing it" (p. 90). Moderators included education, sources of information, and religiosity. Participants were randomized into the control arm, intervention provided to the patient only, or intervention provided to the patient and

a family member. The intervention was delivered weekly for eight weeks. Measures were taken at baseline and at four and seven months using an investigator-developed checklist as well as two additional scales. Change in cancer knowledge was modified by education. Participants with low education who received the patient and family member intervention benefited more than controls and had a greater increase in knowledge from baseline to the four-month measure. Education was not found to moderate patient-provider communication. Extrinsic religiosity was found to be a significant moderator of intervention effectiveness in patient-provider communication. The authors concluded that educational interventions need to be applicable to patients who seek support in religion-oriented activities.

Ezer et al. (2006) collected data on 70 wives at the time their husbands were diagnosed with prostate cancer and three months later. The authors sought to test their model of family adaptation theory to examine whether symptom distress, personal and family resources, and situational appraisal were predictors of adaptation at time point one (T1) and time point two (T2). They also wanted to verify if appraisal served as a mediator at both time points and, finally, to see if predictor variables between the time points would explain the wives' adaptation at T2 and change in adaptation at T1 and T2. A variety of instruments were used for measurement. Testing the model with selected variables explained 30%–50% of the variance in global adaptation and 47%–63% of the variance in emotional adaptation. The variables were a strong predictor of the Profile of Mood States score and a moderate to strong predictor for the Psychosocial Adjustment to Illness Scale–Spouse Version. Sense of coherence (SOC) was the strongest and most consistent predictor in the model for adaptation and was measured with the Antonovsky SOC scale. Researchers found family resources to not be mobilized early on and to be an important predictor of mood at T2. Although some differences are noted at T1 and T2, leading the researchers to question the stability of the model, the authors provided both clinical recommendations based on women's SOC and future directions for interventional study.

In a study of 263 patient-spouse dyads, Northouse et al. (2007) examined the impact of phases of illness on QOL, appraisal of illness, resources, symptoms, and risk for distress. The three phases of treatment identified were newly diagnosed (n = 170), biochemical recurrence (n = 33), and advanced disease (n = 60). Methods included a variety of instruments to gather data. The dyads with advanced disease were found to have significantly (p < .001) poorer physical, emotional, functional and total QOL compared to newly diagnosed dyads. Additionally, patients with advanced disease had significantly (p < .001) lower scores on physical QOL and higher emotional QOL (p < .001) than their spouses. Negative appraisal of illness and caregiving were both reported more in advanced and biochemical dyads, as were hopelessness and uncertainty, with wives having uncertainty. Self-efficacy was higher in those newly diagnosed, and patients were found to report more self-efficacy and social support than their wives. Patients with advanced disease reported more symptom distress and were at higher risk for distress. All patients reported more symptom distress than their wives, as would be expected as symptoms varied based on the patient's phase. Newly diagnosed dyads with patients undergoing prostatectomy were found to have lower social well-being (patient p < .01; wife p < .01) and worse urinary (p < .001) and sexual problems (p < .001) but fewer bowel problems (p < .001) than patients receiving RT. The researchers concluded that phase of illness has more of an impact than role, and both the patient and spouse are affected. Future research and clinical programs should focus on the phase of illness and the interventions that may be warranted.

The final study in this section reviewed the challenges of accrual and retention of subjects in a longitudinal interventional study of families (Northouse et al., 2006). The authors reported on the issues surrounding recruitment and retention as well as strategies that they found to be effective. This study relates to the same parent study as the prior study. In the parent study, 429 dyads were referred to the study, with a final sample size of 218 dyads that completed four measurement time points over 12 months. The researchers found that of those referred, 27.7% were deemed ineligible and another 77.3% of those who were eligible refused, most frequently because they were not interested or were too busy. More patients than spouses reported being not interested (p < .001). Retention at the three sites was 82.9%, and attrition was noted to be highest between the first two measures and higher in the intervention group. The top three reasons for study withdrawal were patient death (33%), declined intervention group (20%), and too busy (13.3%). Staffing factors that affected accrual included workload acuity and the amount of time needed to contact dyads. Retention issues were most obviously affected by phase of illness. Dyads in the newly diagnosed phase were more likely to withdraw because of intervention or the questionnaires, whereas patients in the biochemical relapse or advanced disease group were more likely to withdraw because of health problems, disease progression, or death. Dyads with more symptom distress, lower QOL, advanced disease, and more uncertainty also were less likely to complete the study. This article provided novice and expert researchers with many practical considerations to incorporate into study design and methodology.

Late Effects and Long-Term Survivorship

With 42% of male cancer survivors having a diagnosis of prostate cancer (National Cancer Institute, 2007), healthcare providers must understand the physical and psychosocial factors affecting survivors as well as how treatment has affected long-term QOL. In the first study, Willener and Hantikainen

(2005) explored individual QOL using the Schedule for the Evaluation of Individual QOL: A Direct Weighting Procedure (SEIQoL-DW) and interviews with 11 men who had undergone radical prostatectomy three to four months earlier. In their study, they found health, family, and relationship with partner to be the three areas that had the most impact on QOL and that relationship with the partner was more important than sexuality. The article profiled three of the participants and how they rated their satisfaction and importance within their top five main categories. This study is the first to use the SEIQoL-DW, and further exploration with this tool should be considered.

The role of complementary and alternative medicine (CAM) in cancer care can be studied across the care continuum. Jones et al. (2007) used a mixed-method approach with 14 African American men to explore their attitudes and cultural beliefs on the use of CAM. All men had completed treatment for prostate cancer. Four themes were identified. The first theme, Importance of Spiritual Needs as CAM modality to health, had two categories: *Importance of Faith in God*, and *God Works Through Healthcare Providers*. All men believed that faith in God helps in the management of prostate cancer. Men described faith to be a coping mechanism and that God alone would not cure their cancer. The second theme, *Value of Education in Relation to CAM*, identified that only two of the participants had used CAM (meditation and herbs). Many of the men voiced that CAM treatments were supernatural, superstitious, and not scientifically proven. The next theme, *Importance of Trust in Selected Healthcare Provider*, described how men believed in God but would still receive medical care. God, spirituality, and religion were seen as a complement to treatment, not as the sole intervention. In the final theme identified, *How Men Decide on What to Believe About CAM Modalities*, all men had an opinion about CAM. Five shared that CAM might help them, whereas eight thought these treatments were shams (excluding prayer), and some were unsure if CAM treatments would help. The one patient using herbs feared ridicule and therefore delayed telling his physician about using them. This study identified the impact of beliefs and prostate cancer survivor perspectives on the use of CAM.

Long-term intimacy needs and concerns were the focus of another article in the literature (Sanders, Pedro, Bantum, & Galbraith, 2006). These researchers conducted focus groups with 10 couples over the course of three time points. The first and third sessions had the couples together, and the second session had the men and women separated. Each focus group had its own theme, and men were anywhere from 1.5–8 years out of treatment. Women and men reported different perspectives (see Table 7-2) related to their relationship. Women noted that their role changed from being protected to providing emotional caregiving and trying not to worry about the situation. From a sexual standpoint, women felt unattractive and unwanted, and a decrease in affection from men was noted because of ex-

Table 7-2. Exemplars of Verbatim Comments Demonstrating Differences Between Men's and Women's Perspectives on Communication, Intimacy, and Relationships

Men	Women
We play macho, but don't kid yourself, we depend on this lady, and if she's not in the equation, we're lost.	As women we buck up and take care of business . . . walking a line being genuinely concerned . . . but not breaking out and making him unduly alarmed.
You know, I would be more inclined to reading. . . . So, reading material that I can take home to help me understand . . . I would react better than face to face.	I mean, us women really enjoy getting together. We can communicate really well and share, you know, but men may not be comfortable with that.
Between work and everything else, I really didn't have a whole lot of time to think about it.	I think that was such a giant aspect of what we all go through. . . . If we had just talked about sex.
[The urologist] raised some of those questions, and when I answered and my wife answered differently, I thought, 'Huh?' I thought we were talking, and we really weren't.	My husband is a private individual even though we have been married 53 years. Men don't communicate about themselves. They are not in tune with their bodies.
I have never felt like I've been sick, and it's never worried me.	I don't think he would have done anything about it. It was like denial. . . . They didn't want to do any surgery, but I insisted something should be done.
The negative surprise is the lack of spontaneity. . . . Guys are used to being able to have mind over matter and to be able to force themselves to produce like they could before.	We should remember you are never too old to have a date night. . . . It just means enjoying each other. . . . It doesn't have to be the full thing.
The lack of spontaneity bothered me a lot. It bothered me more than I thought it would at the time.	It's made us different as a couple. . . . The sex has to be different . . . and I decided to make me feel like him . . . less sexual.
From diagnosis to surgery, I was literally paralyzed with fear. . . . After surgery, I kept myself busy.	Our roles are changing. He used to be my protector; now, all of a sudden, I'm protecting him and taking care of him, and it's kinda odd.

Note. From "Couples Surviving Prostate Cancer: Long-Term Intimacy Needs and Concerns Following Treatment," by S. Sanders, L.W. Pedro, E.O. Bantum, and M.E. Galbraith, *Clinical Journal of Oncology Nursing, 10*(4), p. 506. Copyright 2006 by Oncology Nursing Society. Reprinted with permission.

pectations related to sexual performance, whereas men stated that sex was less romantic and more difficult. Both sexes said that too much preparation and planning was involved, with no spontaneity. Women noted a lack of sexual information, and both sexes reported communication challenges. This study identified that couples need more information, yet how wives and husbands want the information delivered may be different. Finally, more open discussion with healthcare providers needs to occur instead of just providing couples with a list of resources.

The last two studies in this topic area explored the impact of two different types of radiation treatments on men's QOL. In the first study, Ward-Smith (2003) used a phenomenologic approach to describe the impact of brachytherapy on QOL in seven men. Five themes were identified, the first being *Post-Treatment Physical Functioning*. This theme identified the changes related to physical functioning, including bladder, bowel, and sexual changes. Negative comments were associated with statements that clarified the impact on QOL; men noted the impact on work and in sexual function.

The next theme, *Treatment Choices and Decision Making*, identified that pamphlets were the most frequently noted education tool. Men also described how they decided upon their treatment choice. Some men made their choice based on it being the least life disruptive, whereas for others, insurance and the inability to undergo surgery were factors. The third theme, *Knowledge of the Disease*, identified that none of the men in this study knew others who had undergone brachytherapy but knew others who had side effects from other treatments. One participant also said that this was a new treatment, and why do something "old-fashioned"? The next theme, *Receiving the Diagnosis*, identified that all men had been diagnosed with a PSA test as part of their annual physical. Men were noted to be extremely knowledgeable about their PSA results and that these values corresponded to diagnosis and treatment. The final theme, *Medication Available Post-Treatment*, stated that all men were offered sildenafil citrate (Viagra®, Pfizer Inc.). Additionally, adherence was an issue with alpha-blocker medications used to decrease urinary hesitancy.

The final study in this area followed 59 men who received external beam RT, with QOL measures taken pretreatment and at 3, 6, and 12 months after treatment (Ward-Smith & Kapitan, 2005). The men completed the 39-item FACT-P instrument, which has five subscales. Three of the five subscales demonstrated statistically significant differences, including the physical well-being subscale (p = .002), the social well-being subscale (p = 0.000), and the prostate concerns subscale (p = .023). Interestingly, the prostate concerns subscale was only significantly different between the pretreatment and three-month post-treatment measure. The impact of treatment was noted across all measurement points of physical well-being and never returned to baseline, whereas emotional and functional well-being mean scores were actually higher at 12 months than they were at baseline. The two subscales most affected provided insight into what it is that nurses need to teach patients as they weigh treatment options, as well as areas of interventional research.

Gaps in the Literature

Many of the studies reviewed in this chapter focused on screening through treatment. Studies related to cancer prevention by nursing researchers were not found, and this may be the result of a variety of factors, including cost, time, and the sample size that might be needed to conduct such a study. Interventional studies focusing on symptom management related to therapy also were not found. Additionally, many of the studies focused on men with localized disease. The need for studies that address men with advanced disease as well as end-of-life care in this population is critical.

Future Directions

Many opportunities lie ahead for nursing researchers in this area. A variety of studies reviewed in this chapter identified communication as an issue that has multiple avenues. Researchers may investigate the role of healthcare provider communication in relation to care and treatment, as well as symptom concerns. This area also is an important one to consider with the role that primary care providers play in patients who require screening. Educational interventions related to hereditary cancer awareness, sexuality, and different methodologies regarding education should continue to be explored.

Nurses need to further investigate family and the relationship changes that arise when a man is diagnosed with prostate cancer, as well as the role of watchful waiting. From the few studies reviewed here, the impact of the diagnosis on the partner may be different and may require a different level of intervention. Additionally, men who are diagnosed in their 40s and 50s who have young or young adult children also should be included in studies related to screening and education. Finally, studies should explore the role of nurses in providing care to this population and the communication and educational resources used to enhance care. Understanding how nurse-led primary care and symptom and survivorship clinics affect screening through end-of-life care is critical to this population.

Conclusion

This chapter provides an overview of nursing contributions to the research literature that focuses on patients with a diagnosis of prostate cancer. The mixture of qualitative and quantitative studies provides the reader with a different way to focus the lens and gather information related to prostate cancer that is not just related to statistical values; rather, it tells a story that will be important in the development of future studies. The studies provide cultural diversity as well as diversity in study methodology.

As the continuum of care evolves and healthcare professionals learn more about prevention and screening, treatment, and symptom management, the role of nursing research will be pivotal in advancing the care of this population. Nursing studies that are outcome driven and that enhance current screening methods, as well as studies that identify opportunities for implementation into practice, are critical. Nurses interact with these patients and their families throughout the continuum of care and therefore need to advocate for, partner with, and promote the science of nursing as this body of literature continues to grow.

References

Davison, B.J., Goldenberg, S.L., Wiens, K.P., & Gleave, M.E. (2007). Comparing a generic and individualized information decision support intervention for men newly diagnosed with localized prostate cancer. *Cancer Nursing, 30*(5), E7–E15. Retrieved January 8, 2008, from http://ovidsp.tx.orvid.com/spb/ovidweb.cgi

Davison, B.J., Moore, K.N., MacMillan, H., Bisaillon, A., & Wiens, K. (2004). Patient evaluation of a discharge program following a radical prostatectomy. *Urologic Nursing, 24*(6), 483–489.

Ezer, H., Ricard, N., Bouchard, L., Souhami, L., Saad, F., Aprikian, A., et al. (2006). Adaptation of wives to prostate cancer following diagnosis and 3 months after treatment: A test of family adaptation theory. *International Journal of Nursing Studies, 43*(7), 827–838.

Hedestig, O., Sandman, P.O., Tomic, R., & Widmark, A. (2005). Living after external beam radiotherapy of localized prostate cancer. *Cancer Nursing, 28*(4), 310–317.

Hedestig, O., Sandman, P.O., & Widmark, A. (2003). Living with untreated localized prostate cancer. *Cancer Nursing, 26*(1), 55–60.

Ilic, D., O'Connor, D., Green, S., & Wilt, T. (2006). Screening for prostate cancer. *Cochrane Database of Systematic Reviews* 2006, Issue 3. Art. No.: CD004720. DOI: 10.1002/14651858.CD004720.pub2.

Institute of Medicine. (2007). *Cancer care for the whole patient: Meeting psychosocial health needs.* Washington, DC: National Academies Press.

Jones, R.A., Taylor, A.G., Bourguignon, C., Steeves, R., Fraser, G., Lippert, M., et al. (2007). Complementary and alternative medicine modality use and beliefs among African American prostate cancer survivors. *Oncology Nursing Forum, 34*(2), 359–364.

Kleier, J.A. (2006). Language adaptation and testing of the prostate health questionnaire for Jamaican and Haitian men. *Urologic Nursing, 26*(4), 304–310.

Meade, C.D., Calvo, A., Rivera, M.A., & Baer, R.D. (2003). Focus groups in the design of prostate cancer screening information for Hispanic farmworkers and African American men. *Oncology Nursing Forum, 30*(6), 967–975.

Mishel, M.H., Germino, B.B., Belyea, M., Stewart, J.L., Bailey, D.E., Jr., Mohler, J., et al. (2003). Moderators of an uncertainty intervention. *Nursing Research, 52*(2), 89–97.

National Cancer Institute. (2007, July 3). *Cancer survivorship research: Estimated U.S. cancer prevalence.* Retrieved September 21, 2007, from http://dccps.nci.nih.gov/ocs/prevalence/prevalence.html#male

Ng, C., Kristjanson, L.J., & Medigovich, K. (2006). Hormone ablation for the treatment of prostate cancer: The lived experience. *Urologic Nursing, 26*(3), 204–212.

Northouse, L.L., Rosset, T., Phillips, L., Mood, D., Schafenacker, A., & Kershaw, T. (2006). Research with families facing cancer: The challenges of accrual and retention. *Research in Nursing and in Health, 29*(3), 199–211.

Northouse, L.L., Mood, D.W., Montie, J.E., Sandler, H.M., Forman, J.D., Hussain, M., et al. (2007). Living with prostate cancer: Patients' and spouses' psychosocial status and quality of life. *Journal of Clinical Oncology, 25*(27), 4171–4177.

Oliffe, J. (2004). Transrectal ultrasound prostate biopsy (TRUS-Bx): Patient perspectives. *Urologic Nursing, 24*(5), 395–400.

Oliffe, J. (2006). Being screened for prostate cancer: A simple blood test or a commitment to treatment? *Cancer Nursing, 29*(1), 1–8.

Oncology Nursing Society. (2005). *Oncology Nursing Society 2005–2009 research agenda talking points.* Retrieved September 21, 2007, from http://www.ons.org/research/information/documents/pdfs/talking05.pdf

Sanders, S., Pedro, L.W., Bantum, E.O., & Galbraith, M.E. (2006). Couples surviving prostate cancer: Long-term intimacy needs and concerns following treatment. *Clinical Journal of Oncology Nursing, 10*(4), 503–508.

Templeton, H., & Coates, V. (2004). Evaluation of an evidence-based education package for men with prostate cancer on hormonal manipulation therapy. *Patient Education and Counseling, 55*(1), 55–61.

Templeton, H.R., & Coates, V.E. (2001). Adaptation of an instrument to measure the informational needs of men with prostate cancer. *Journal of Advanced Nursing, 35*(3), 357–364.

Ward-Smith, P. (2003). Brachytherapy for prostate cancer: The patient's perspective. *Urologic Nursing, 23*(3), 213–217.

Ward-Smith, P., & Kapitan, D. (2005). Quality of life among men treated with radiation therapy for prostate cancer. *Urologic Nursing, 25*(4), 263–268.

Weinrich, S., Vijayakumar, S., Powell, I.J., Priest, J., Hamner, C.A., McCloud, L., et al. (2007). Knowledge of hereditary prostate cancer among high-risk African American men. *Oncology Nursing Forum, 34*(4), 854–860.

Weinrich, S.P., Seger, R., Curtsinger, T., Pumphrey, G., NeSmither, E.G., & Weinrich, M.C. (2007). Impact of pretest on posttest knowledge scores with a Solomon Four research design. *Cancer Nursing, 30*(5), E16–E28. Retrieved January 8, 2008, from http://ovidsp.tx.ovid.com/spb/ovidweb.cgi

Willener, R., & Hantikainen, V. (2005). Individual quality of life following radical prostatectomy in men with prostate cancer. *Urologic Nursing, 25*(2), 88–100.

Wettergren, L., Björkholm, M., & Langius-Eklöf, A. (2005). Validation of an extended version of the SEIQoL-DW in a cohort of Hodgkin lymphoma survivors. *Quality of Life Research, 14*(10), 2329–2333.

Index

The letter f after a page number indicates that relevant content appears in a figure; the letter t, in a table.

urinary symptoms, 4, 8, 40, 59,
69, 71*t*–72*t*, 95
Us TOO International Prostate
Cancer Education and
Support Network, 1, 99*t*

V

vaccine therapy, 44

vacuum constriction device,
78*t*, 89
vardenafil, 78*t*
venlafaxine, 57, 88
vinorelbine, 62
vitamin A, 24
vitamin D, 88
vitamin E, 24, 26
vitamin supplementation, 69–70
vomiting, 64*t*

W

Ware Health Perceptions
Questionnaire, 100*f*
watchful waiting, 35–36, 36*f*,
55–56, 98, 107
weight gain, 90
wellness care, 101
Wellness Community, 99*t*
workplace concerns, 98

World Health Organization
(WHO), 61, 87

Z

zoledronic acid, 39–40, 77,
79–80